Body Image and Disfigurement Care

Body Image and Disfigurement Care is intended for use by all health care professionals working with patients who have suffered a threat to body image, whether from trauma, injury, disease, or the developmental process. This book:

- offers practical advice about care
- critically appraises the existing knowledge-base
- describes the different theoretical approaches to body image disturbance
- puts forward a new model of what happens to people with disturbed body image.

While written in an accessible style, this is not a superficial text. It presents practical skills, based on appropriate research evidence, which can be used in clinical settings. Interactive exercises enable students to consolidate their learning and improve their understanding of the patient's experience of a threat to body image.

Body Image and Disfigurement Care provides a sound source of help and advice about an issue of growing importance in modern health care.

Robert Newell is Senior Lecturer in the School of Healthcare Studies, University of Leeds.

Routledge Essentials for Nurses

Series editors: Robert Newell, *University of Leeds*, and David Thompson, *University of York*

Routledge Essentials for Nurses cover four key areas of nursing:

- core theoretical studies
- psychological and physical care
- nurse education
- new directions in nursing and health care

Written by experienced practitioners and teachers, books in the series encourage a critical approach to nursing concepts and show how research findings are relevant to nursing practice.

Nursing Theories and Models
Hugh McKenna

Nursing Perspectives on Quality of Life
Peter Draper

Education for Patients and Clients
Vivien Coates

Caring for People in Pain
Bryn D. Davis

Body Image and Disfigurement Care
Robert Newell

Design and Analysis of Clinical Nursing Research Studies
Colin R. Martin and David R. Thompson

Sociology and Nursing
Peter Morrall

Body Image and Disfigurement Care

Robert Newell

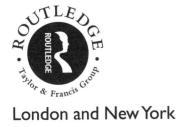

London and New York

First published 2000
by Routledge
11 New Fetter Lane, London EC4P 4EE

Simultaneously published in the USA and Canada
by Routledge
29 West 35th Street, New York, NY 10001

Routledge is an imprint of the Taylor & Francis Group

Typeset in Times and Gill Sans by
Prepress Projects Ltd, Perth, Scotland
Printed and bound in Great Britain by
Clays Ltd, St Ives, plc

British Library Cataloguing in Publication Data
A catalogue record for this book is available
from the British Library

Library of Congress Cataloging in Publication Data
Newell, Robert, 1954–
    Body image and disfigurement care / Robert Newell.
    p.   cm. –
    Includes bibliographical references and index.
    ISBN 0-415-22596-5 (HB) – ISBN 0-415-22597-3 (PB)
    1. Disfigured persons – Rehabilitation. 2. Cognitive therapy. 3.
    Body image.
    I. Title. II. Series.
    [DNLM: 1. Abnormalities – psychology. 2. Body Image. 3.
    Cognition Disorders – psychology. 4. Cognitive Therapy. 5. Facial
    Injuries – psychology. 6. Wounds and Injuries – psychology. WM
    204 N546b 2000]
    RD761 .N49 2000
    616.89–dc21   00-032187

To Caroline

Contents

Illustrations

Chapter 1

Introduction

The nature of body image and disfigurement

We all form and retain images of our bodies. During our lives these body images go through many changes, some of which are desired, whilst others are not. For example, we attempt to alter the way our bodies look, perhaps out of a desire to express our individuality or to conform with commonly perceived norms of excellence of bodily appearance. Indeed, the cosmetics, fashion, sports and leisure industries are greatly concerned with the building and maintenance of these norms, which they then service through a range of products. At one extreme, aesthetic plastic surgery (cosmetic surgery) involves comparatively permanent changes to bodily appearance, through which people seek to achieve a desired appearance.

By contrast, some changes in bodily appearance, and associated changes in body image, are not desired. Whether from birth, through trauma or disease or as a result of the ageing process, certain aspects of bodily appearance are almost universally regarded as unwanted by those people who have received them. These changes in appearance and body image have received considerable attention in the nursing and medical literature, but there has been, surprisingly, comparatively little study of the experiences of those who have undergone changes to physical appearance, their adjustment to these changes, attempts to address their difficulties, or the reactions of others to them. Whilst some areas (for example breast cancer, anorexia nervosa) have received rather more coverage than others, there are many complaints for which issues of body image are much less frequently discussed, still less empirically studied. Moreover, in many cases, the focus of the study is on the *illness* which is associated with the changes to the body. Whilst this may seem natural, it is debatable how much such studies tell us about the relationship between changes to the body's appearance and function, on the one hand, and body image and its disturbance, on the other. This is because disease-specific studies are often concerned not just with changes in appearance and function, but also with many other issues, such as the experience of being diagnosed with and living with a life-threatening illness, and the practical consequences of altered bodily functions.

Nevertheless, many people with altered body appearance and function are *not suffering from any illness*. It is part of the intention of this book to argue that the best approach to their difficulties is to examine responses to altered bodily appearance and function chiefly as issues or problems in their own right, rather than as add-ons to some disease process. Consider the burns survivor, the diabetic person, the person who has undergone amputation, the cancer patient no longer receiving treatment and 'in remission'. For some purposes, it will certainly be relevant to consider them in the context of the event which gave rise to changes in their appearance. However, this book argues two things: first, that these individuals are not primarily (or even actually) patients – they are simply people who have a potential for difficulties related to body image; second, that an approach which examines the life problems of people experiencing a challenge to body image outside of the context of disease or illness is a useful way of addressing such difficulties. Appeals to disease and illness are not required except where these have a clear contribution to make to our understanding of these difficulties.

The aims of the book

This book puts forward a general model of what might be going on in body image, changes to body image following threat and ways of addressing any difficulties which may result. This model of body image and its disturbance (the fear–avoidance model) is neither disease specific, nor illness based, but is based on a particular cognitive-behavioural approach to human experience and behaviour. Whilst the detailed examination of this model and the predictions it makes about human behaviour following challenges to body image are undertaken in Chapters 3 and 8, its basic tenets can be summarised as follows:

- the model is based on cognitive and conditioning accounts of human experience and behaviour
- the model attempts to differentiate between those who experience difficulty and those who do not following challenges to body image
- the model attempts to predict what interventions might be helpful.

This approach was principally developed with people who have experienced a facial disfigurement (Newell 1999), regardless of diagnosis. It is suggested here that the approach has wider application, and a considerable number of suggestions about such application will be made in this book. Moreover, similar approaches have proved robust across a number of client difficulties, from phobias (Marks 1987) to chronic pain states (Lethem *et al.* 1983; Rose *et al.* 1992).

However, the major focus of this book will be upon disfigurement in general, and facial disfigurement in particular. There are many threats to body image which are *not* visible, such as loss or damage to internal body organs or the intrusion of artificial or transplanted body parts. Disfigurement, however, possesses particular characteristics which make it especially useful for a consideration of body image. Firstly, there is no reason to suppose that all the elements of threat to body image which are present in non-visible bodily changes are not also present in visible ones. For example, we have no reason to suppose that reactions to a visible prosthetic will be less far-reaching than those to an invisible one. Indeed, we might suppose the reverse, since the additional characteristic of visibility will be possessed in the former case. This notion of visibility is important, since it bears on stigma. Stigmata were originally *visible* marks of slavery by which an enslaved person's status was known to others. Goffman (1963) draws the distinction between discredited and discreditable stigmatised people. Discredited persons are unable to hide the attributes which give rise to their stigmatised status, whilst discreditable people would be stigmatised if such attributes were visible, but are able to hide them. In most situations, disfigured people are unable to hide their disfigurements (although, as we shall see in Chapter 7, considerable effort is often put into attempting to do so), and thus may be thought to bear the additional burden of stigma from other people. Focusing on disfigurement allows us to examine the impact of stigma. We shall also examine (in Chapter 3) the possibility that continuing exposure to stigmatising situations may actually be *helpful*, by promoting adaptation in the manner suggested by Newell (1991) and Dropkin (1989). Finally, disfigured people are, in many ways, the example *par excellence* of well people who are experiencing a severe challenge to body image, since many (burn survivors, traumatic injury survivors, people with birth defects) have no continuing physical illness. For this reason, we can be relatively confident that, in many cases, the difficulties they experience are the result of body image disturbance, rather than of such factors as fear of ongoing treatment, illness or disability. Moreover, for facially disfigured people, there are often few of the practical difficulties associated with amputations or with the removal of functioning organs, with the sole exception that presentation of the self is mediated to a considerable degree by the face, and such self-presentation is itself an exceedingly important function. Self-presentation, however, is not limited to the face, and the role of self-presentation in adaptation to challenges to body image is examined in Chapter 2.

In summary, then, facial disfigurement is an ideal example to draw upon in our examination of body image and its disturbance, particularly in the context of exploring body image challenges in well people. It is the contention of this text that, if the issues surrounding this example are fully explored by the reader, a considerable amount of generally applicable information can be gained which will be useful in addressing challenges to body image in a wide range of patient groups.

The structure of the book

The fear–avoidance model has its origins in clinical practice, but also in the body of work which precedes it in the area of disfigurement, and in approaches to body image from a mental health and illness perspective. The structure of this book reflects this background, by commencing with an examination in Chapter 2 of several of the major current models of body image disturbance. This chapter also sets the scene for much of the rest of the book by touching on the history of our understanding of body image and on issues of measurement of body image. This material informs much of the content of Chapter 3, which lays out the cognitive-behavioural approach which forms the basis for the therapeutic approach suggested later.

Part 2 begins with, in Chapter 4, a broad examination of stigma, with particular reference to its potential effect on body image disturbance. Stigma is often regarded as crucial in the development of social difficulties amongst disfigured people in particular, and disabled people in general, and has informed many of the empirical studies of social interactions with such individuals. These studies are examined in Chapters 5 and 6. Qualitative research has been of considerable importance in mapping the territory with regard to the experiences of disfigured people, and provides an invaluable insight into these experiences. This work has more recently been complemented by attempts to apply a more structured, generalisable approach to the examination of such experiences, and relevant quantitative studies are examined. In Chapter 6, we turn to attempts to ameliorate the difficulties of disfigured people in particular, once again using facial disfigurement as the critical case example for application to body image disturbance. Selected studies from fields other than facial disfigurement are also examined, in order to complement the examination of studies of disfigured people. In essence, Part 2 provides the empirical research background which informs the fear–avoidance approach.

Part 3 examines this approach more directly and attempts to apply this information to practice. Thus, in Chapter 7, a number of recent attempts (Newell 1998, 1999, 2000; Newell and Clark 2000; Newell and Marks 2000) to test the model are examined. In each case, the way in which the results of the studies might be said to support the cognitive-behavioural approach is outlined. Chapter 8 attempts to draw conclusions about actual treatment interventions from the rest of the book. The emphasis is placed on the model described in Chapter 3 and the empirical tests outlined in Chapter 7. This final chapter aims both to present the reader with a series of possible strategies to be employed during interventions with people who have suffered a disturbance in body image and also to demonstrate a rationale for the use of such interventions which is, as far as possible given the relatively immature state of the area, based upon evidence.

The future

The elements of this book which relate to the fear–avoidance model and the cognitive-behavioural approach derived from it are under continuing development. As a consequence, this book is, itself, still a work in progress. In Chapter 8, some of the work still to be done with regard both to interventions with disturbed body image in general and to the cognitive-behavioural approach in particular is outlined. It should be noted at the outset, however, that readers of this book are also, I hope, potential contributors to endeavours to offer a focused, evidence-based approach to the difficulties of people who have experienced a change in physical appearance and body image. This book attempts to present an approach which will have general applicability and become evidence based. This evidence base is still in its infancy. Indeed, Francis Macgregor, who has worked in the field of facial disfigurement for nearly 50 years, has repeatedly stressed the need to add to the impoverished research base of this topic. If readers of this book use the tactics offered here, I would welcome hearing about their results. It is essential that interventions with people who have experienced changes in body image are rigorously evaluated. I will also welcome discussion with readers over potential ways to effect such evaluations.

A note on gender: Where no particular gender is implied by the context, the female personal pronoun is used, to reflect the role of women as the greater providers and recipients of health care.

A note on study participation: In general, the term 'participant' has come to be favoured over 'subject' when describing individuals whose responses are examined as part of a study, even though there is slight inaccuracy here since the researcher is also a study participant. However, this usage is retained in this book for general descriptive purposes. Where specific studies are examined, the term used by the study authors is retained.

Part I

Approaches to body image

Chapter 2

Elements of body image

The need for models of body image

Nursing as an activity is intimately concerned with the body's appearance and functions, including the most intimate aspects of these appearances and functions. If we consider the activities of caring, a great many of these are concerned either with intimate personal services such as washing, bathing and helping with toileting or with clinical procedures which involve exposing parts of the body which would not normally be exposed in the ordinary social context and intruding upon the body in unusual ways. As nurses, we are given privileged access to patients' bodies by virtue of our clinical role.

This privileged access carries with it the responsibility of behaving professionally during intimate procedures, since such professional behaviour is necessary to preserve the dignity of the patient. It is, however, far from obvious what we might mean by professional behaviour in this context. At one level, we might think about preserving an appropriately formal distance from the patient, and it is probably clear that we are aware of what breaches of such distance amount to, since they are enshrined in our culture in knockabout film comedy and seaside post cards. However, such distance should not deny the fact that we all have bodies and respond to the bodily appearance and functions of others, often in complex ways. Indeed, there are many situations where the preservation of professional aloofness is clearly antitherapeutic, and probably designed more to protect the nurse from embarrassment or other responses to issues about her own body than to protect the patient from unwanted intrusion outside the relationship of professional privilege.

It is easy to generate examples of where such 'antitherapeutic' behaviour may occur. If a nurse is uncomfortable with her own body and with intimate contact with others, we may expect her physical handling to demonstrate elements of that tension. Similarly, if she is uncomfortable about discussing matters of intimate appearance or function, we may expect that such discussion will be stilted, or even absent, and that the patient will be unlikely to voice any concerns she may have. Whilst it is a given in our society that people are more comfortable about their bodies and sexuality than, say, 20 years ago, the limits of that comfort are explored and tested daily in health care generally, and in nursing in particular. As an experiment, consider how happy you would feel if, in the interests of experiential learning, you were required to role play being given an intramuscular injection into the exposed buttock, possibly from a member of the opposite sex, separated from a roomful of people by only a thin curtain. To my knowledge, we do not require student nurses to undergo such experiences during training, but I predict that there would be considerable disquiet from such students if we introduced such an initiative. It may be instructive to consider the likely range of excuses for non-participation. Yet such a procedure is a relatively innocuous threat to body image.

By contrast, we expect patients to endure such procedures routinely. Which brings us back to the notion of professional behaviour as a way of safeguarding patients' dignity. In the previous paragraphs, I have tried to suggest that bland professional detachment is, at best, a limited definition of professional behaviour and, at worst, antitherapeutic. As an alternative, I suggest that professional behaviour related to intimate contact and discussion with patients lies in our ability to understand the nature of our own and our patients' experiences of the body.

Models of body image are simply descriptive attempts to explain these experiences, be they physical, perceptual or behavioural. They are useful to us because they attempt to increase our understanding of body image, principally through organising complex information in a systematic way. Naturally, much is lost in the process, since models need to simplify the wealth of information available in order to make it comprehensible. One of the tests of a good model is how well it balances the competing needs to simplify and to be comprehensive. I do not propose to dwell on the nature of models in nursing, and interested readers are directed to Hugh McKenna's (1997) excellent book in this series. It is, however, useful to think of a model as a kind of conceptual map or diagram. No one would ever confuse a map of the Peak District National Park with the *actual* Peak District nor a diagram of the heart in a physiology book with an *actual* heart. There are, apart from differences of scale, many omissions – there are no trees drawn on maps of the peaks, no blood drawn in the heart, no representation of people on the maps, no accuracy of colour in the diagram, and so on. Similarly, no model can be truly comprehensive and we may need different models for different purposes, in the same way different maps are used for travel, mountaineering, political purposes, weather, and so on.

Despite this, the value of these representations lies in the accuracy with which they describe (or model) certain characteristics or functions of the entities they purport to represent. From this accuracy comes their ability to aid our understanding. One important element of this is the notion of prediction. A useful model allows us to make and test certain predictions about the entity being modelled. We can, for example, from examining maps of the countryside, attempt to find a route between certain points. If the map is accurate (and our interpretation of it is correct!) we expect to end up at the desired end point. Likewise, a diagram of the heart which did not conform to our observations of bloodflow in an actual heart would be of little value. In both these cases, we ask how far predictions we make based on the model are borne out in real life. If they are not, this represents an important, and possibly critical, flaw in the model.

In many situations, models are rather more complex than diagrams, since the entities they seek to examine are also complex. However, the general point remains that models should accurately describe some dimension or dimensions of the thing they purport to. Part of the notion of accuracy is the ability to predict the behaviour of the actual entity from the model. In the case of body image, a successful model has to account for a broad range of often complex behaviours. During the past 60 years or so, some efforts have been made towards definitions of body image, although, surprisingly for a profession so closely concerned with the body, little of this work has come from nursing, with the important exceptions of Price in the UK and Dropkin in the USA. Moreover, such models as do exist are not without their difficulties. In the remainder of this chapter, we shall trace the development of the concept of body image, and examine three major approaches to that concept.

The concept of body image

Body image is central to the consideration of appearance and disfigurement even when it is not explicitly identified. For example, studies of attractiveness suggest that people carry common concepts of what constitutes attractiveness, the psychological attributes which accompany attractiveness, and the appropriate ways of behaving towards more and less attractive people. In facial disfigurement, it appears that preferences for non-disfigured individuals are learnt early in life and demonstrable across a wide range of situations, again suggesting abiding shared attitudes about what constitutes acceptable and unacceptable appearance. The difficulties experienced by disfigured people may represent a mismatch between their appearance and that shared perception of what is acceptable, a perception which they themselves share. In Price's (1990a, 1990b) model, explored later in this chapter, this represents a mismatch between the body ideal and body reality components of body image.

Although numerous commentators agree that body image as an expression has often been used in a loose, ill-defined way (Lacey and Birchnell 1986; Cumming 1988; Brown *et al.* 1990), it is generally agreed that the term is separate from, although related to, such concepts as self-image, self-esteem and self-concept (Dewing 1989). None of these broader terms are explored in this text. Schilder (1935) defines body image as 'The picture of our body which we form in our mind, that is to say the way in which our body appears to ourselves', a definition which has remained as the starting point for later conceptualisations of body image until today. He also describes body image as a 'tri-dimensional image every body has about himself'. For much of his writing, Schilder (1935) uses the term body image interchangeably to apply to physical perception of the body and psychological attitudes to it. His major contribution to the definition of body image is, however, the incorporation of these attitudinal aspects, and his drawing of a distinction between these aspects and physical perception. As we shall see later, at least one major writer in the field has, however, suggested that distinctions between perceptual and attitudinal aspects of body image are unlikely to be categorical (Slade 1994). Although the terms are sometimes used interchangeably by Schilder (1935), *body schema* is most often currently used to refer to the perceptual elements of body image, whilst *body image* often includes both these elements and evaluative components (see, for example, Cumming (1988) and Slade (1988)).

Schilder further notes that body image is dynamic, changing both during the life cycle and in response to short-term alterations such as changes of mood or even changes of clothing or the use of instruments such as tools, which extend that image. We can easily see the perceptual aspect of this extension by, for example, our experience of driving a car. Very early in learning to drive, we come to perceive the width of the car without having always to look to each side as we drive, in much the same way that we need not check each side of our bodies when passing through a door. With regard to the attitudinal aspect, the attachments people form to particular items of clothing or jewellery suggest that these have been incorporated into our images of ourselves through becoming an extension of our body images. Indeed, the suggestion that *self* image is primarily physical or bodily can be traced back at least to the writings of Freud (Bronheim *et al.* 1991).

From the psychoanalytical standpoint, Schilder (1935) notes the relationship between attitudinal elements of body image and drives to satisfy basic needs within the body. Similarly, many such attitudes are seen as linked to bodily sensations. It seems that he views bodily sensations, psychological body image and the ego as being intimately related, a view consistent with the Freudian formulation, noted above, of the ego as principally deriving from bodily phenomena. Importantly, however, Schilder goes beyond this view of body image as an internally driven phenomenon in the latter part of his book. Here, he notes that body image is essentially a public phenomenon. According to Schilder, the body image is in a state of continuous construction, destruction and reconstruction by virtue of its reciprocal interaction with the body images of those with whom we come into contact (Schilder 1935). Part of this reciprocity involves the imitation of others, whose body images come to be incorporated within our own, either through integration within or addition to our previous views of ourselves. In his conclusion, Schilder emphasises the relatedness of the somatic, psychological and interactional aspects of body image, thus giving an early bio-psychosocial account of the phenomenon, which is also an analogue of the three systems approach to human difficulties (Lang 1971) outlined later in this book.

As we noted above, Schilder attempted to draw a basic distinction between aspects of body image – the distinction between perception and appraisal or attitude. Cumming (1988) has pointed out that, for practical purposes, the distinction refers to whether we are considering body image in a neurological or in a psychological sense. In the first instance, we are talking of perceptual facts, whilst in the second, we are describing subjective experiences. Naturally, this is an incomplete distinction, which Schilder acknowledged in his description of the reciprocity of the somatic, psychological and social elements in body image. For example, neurological disorders which distort our physical appreciation of the body's position, and perhaps alter our control of our movements, will influence our confidence in performing tasks or interacting with others and will affect our satisfaction with our body. Nevertheless, the distinction has been widely applied. In the field of eating disorders, for example, the difference between attitude to body size and misperception of that size is regarded as a key empirical distinction (Keeton *et al.* 1990), with considerable evidence to show that anorexics overestimate body size

(Gardner and Moncrieff 1988), as well as being dissatisfied with that size.

Models of body image

In nursing in the UK, perhaps the clearest and most comprehensive account of body image comes from Price (1990a, 1990b). At the root of his model is a view of body image as consisting of three related components: body reality, body ideal and body presentation (see Figure 2.1).

Price's main examination of the body image which he asserts is made up of these elements is in terms of psychological experiences. However, physical perceptions of the body are not excluded from his model. For Price, *body reality* is the body as it is constructed, and includes both external elements such as height and weight and internal elements such as organs of the body and functions such as digestion or fluid balance. The notion that bodily *functions* are part of our image of the body appears

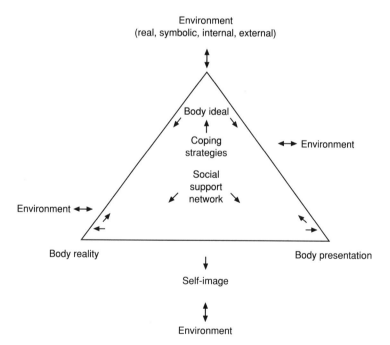

Figure 2.1 Price's model of body image. Arrows indicate direction of influence or interaction (after Price 1990a)

important, particularly in the context of impairment of function, although it is not extensively examined in the body image literature. We might argue that impairment of functioning is as important a threat to body image as disfigured appearance. Moreover, appearance and function are often linked. Finally, appearance is itself a complex social function, whose disturbance has been thought to contribute to negative stereotyping of disfigured people (Macgregor 1990). Elements of body schema, such as awareness of spatial characteristics of the body (Cumming 1988), should by inference be considered as part of body reality in Price's model, since such a schema is itself a bodily function.

Body reality is recognised as being both changeable throughout the life cycle and in immediate response to our interactions with the environment. Naturally, body reality can also change as a result of insults to the body through disease or trauma. The defining characteristic of body reality is that it is not consequent upon our attitudes to it, but consists of physical attributes of the body.

By contrast, *body ideal* is attitudinal, and represents the way we would wish our bodies to be. Like Schilder (1935), Price sees this ideal as being gained through a process of identification with the body ideals of others, as revealed to us through our interactions with the rest of society. Our body ideal might thus be construed as a set of internalised societal norms of how society as a whole thinks we should look and the way in which it thinks our bodies should function. Naturally, as members of that society, we all share these views in some degree and contribute to their construction and modification. Some such views are relatively old and lasting, such as the apparent preference amongst animals for symmetry (see Bernstein (1976) for a note on the applicability of this issue to burns patients) or the preference for 'attractiveness' observed in relatively young children (Rumsey *et al.* 1986a). Others are new, and likely to be transient, and we usually call these fashion, even when they require relatively lasting changes to body reality in order to meet the new ideal, as in the recent trends towards tattooing and artificially constructed scars.

Newell (1991) has noted the behavioural view of how individuals might acquire notions of the body ideal through the process of differential reinforcement of behaviours which reflect attitudes consistent with the prevailing norms of body image. For example, in our everyday experience we see how peer pressure is rewarding for children who have the latest football team strip, the haircut of a favourite film star, and so on. Since it is likely that behaviours themselves affect attitude formation and change (Festinger 1957; Zimbardo and Ebbeson 1970), the reinforcement of behaviours consistent with such norms may then alter people's attitudes, including their *own* body ideals. By contrast, people whose appearance deviates from the attractive body ideal of society are generally sanctioned by the lack of availability of reinforcement opportunities in such diverse aspects of social life as work (e.g. Raza and Carpenter 1987), socialising (Kleck and Rubenstein 1975) and dating (Reis *et al.* 1980). Body ideal appears a largely learnt phenomenon, contingent upon societal definitions of the ideal. It may be influenced by changes in body reality, but is not necessarily matched to this reality. Indeed, according to Price's model, a mismatch between the reality and the ideal may be the cause of considerable personal difficulty.

Finally, *body presentation* refers to how we present all aspects of our bodily appearance, including dress, grooming and behaviour. It is, to a marked extent, under the conscious control of the individual, who may, within limits, alter the presentation of the body reality in the direction of conformity with the ideal.

To these three linked elements, Price (1990a) has added several contributing components which influence them. *Coping strategies* direct how individuals will respond to threats to body image integrity in the context of their *social support network*, which forms part of a more general *influence of environment*. Price also emphasises the related nature of body image and self image. In Price's (1990a, 1990b) descriptions of body image, he sees the three elements as existing in a state of tension or balance which together make up a satisfactory body image which we all strive to maintain. For example, we might suppose that alterations to body reality (for example from surgery or disease) would result in increased tension between that reality and body ideal. As a response to this tension, the individual might attempt to alter body presentation in such a way as to compensate for the deficiency in body reality, or might change their own attitudes to what constitutes their body ideal, invoking particular coping strategies and social supports in order to help make these compensatory changes. These responses might be expected to lead to a decrease in the tension between reality and ideal.

Price's model has considerable appeal and is potentially useful as a way of conceptualising body image, its disturbance and health care responses to that disturbance. As we noted above, the description of the body ideal and its acquisition may be accounted for by appeals to theories of conditioning and attitude change, whilst body reality is apparently comprehensive in its inclusion of bodily attributes and functions. Finally, body presentation as an aspect of body image corresponds to Schilder's description of appearance and behaviour contributing to body image. Thus, Price's model of body image is consistent with descriptions of social learning and is potentially a comprehensive explanation.

However, the ways in which the elements of Price's model might be said to influence each other, and the putative consequences if one or more of the elements are disturbed, are less clear. Price (1990a, 1990b) provides clinical examples of disturbance in body image and its effect with regard to the three elements. He also gives examples of how the elements relate to a model of body image care. However, these examples are basically clinical anecdotes which are designed to illustrate particular aspects of both disturbance and care. Whilst this is useful, it unfortunately gives us no sense of whether they are in any way typical. If they are not, this represents an obvious weakness for the model, and the conclusions we might wish to draw about approaches to patient care would clearly be very limited. Certainly, no systematised empirical examinations of Price's model exist to date. For example, we do not know whether changes in one aspect of body image are causative of changes in another, consequent upon such changes or independent of them. Moreover, it may prove difficult even to operationalise the various elements of Price's model to a sufficient degree to make specific predictions which can then be tested.

The general construction of the model is somewhat circular, with the consequence that prediction of possible responses which might result from its assumptions is difficult. As an example of this circularity, the model lacks an adequate definition of satisfactory body image. The problem with this becomes apparent when Price (1990b) tells us that balancing the three components of body image is a state of well-being or body image health, and, later, that tension and balance between the three elements are necessary to sustain a satisfactory body image. However, what is this satisfactory state which the balance seeks to maintain? Balance itself cannot be sufficient for satisfactory body image, since we could conceive of a person who had a very low body ideal, very poor body reality and very poor body presentation. This individual would have a perfectly balanced body image which we would not describe as being satisfactory.

In the absence of a clear definition of 'satisfactory body image', it is also difficult to argue which behaviours will have either a positive or a negative effect on such an image. A definition of altered body image was added by Price (1996):

> A state of personal distress, defined by the patient, which indicates that the body no longer supports self-esteem, and which is dysfunctional to individuals, limiting their social engagement with others. Altered body image exists when coping strategies (individual

and social) to deal with changes in body reality, ideal or presentation, are overwhelmed by injury, disease, disability or social stigma.

(Price 1996: 170)

This definition is, unfortunately, inadequate in a number of ways. On the one hand, its comprehensivity is insufficient, since we can easily see situations in which body image might be disturbed without the necessity for coping strategies to be overwhelmed (for example, phantom sensations which the individual accepts). On the other, the definition, if necessary at all, does not add any greater clarity to our understanding of the supposed directions of interaction between the components said to comprise body image. It should be noted, however, that the lack of a definition is of importance only if it limits our ability to draw conclusions from a particular model. It may be that a simple definition, such as Goin and Goin's (1981) suggestion that undisturbed body image is that which does not interfere with physical and psychological functioning, is sufficient if it allows us to test such models.

A further problem is caused for Price's model by the fact that both body ideal and body presentation may be capable of change in the face of threats to body image through changes in body reality. Whilst on the one hand it is quite reasonable that both such dimensions of body image should change in this way, it is problematic because it leads to a situation where almost any set of behaviours can be explained by Price's model. This in turn is problematic because such explanations are likely to lack any predictive value, and the consequence of this is that the model may be rendered both theoretically untestable and practically useless. As an example, say an individual's body presentation changes in response to a threatening change in body reality. We might justifiably say he was attempting, through manipulation of body presentation, to narrow an increased discrepancy between ideal and reality resulting from the change in reality. This would support the notion of satisfactory body image relying on balance between the three elements. However, if body presentation did not change, this would not necessarily constitute a refutation of the model, since we could argue that the person had instead modified their body ideal, restoring balance between the three elements in this way.

Both these occurrences may indeed be possible. However, in the absence of tight specification of the circumstances in which attitude rather than behaviour change would be expected, the model possesses the weakness that it does not predict whether behaviour change (or, indeed, attitude change) will occur or not under a given set of circumstances. This diminishes the clinical usefulness of the model, since it is difficult to see how our practice might be guided by a model which does not predict what will happen to patients under particular circumstances. Empirical investigation of Price's model, involving tight specifications and consistent measurement tactics, should now be undertaken.

This is not to say that Price's (1990a, 1990b) model is unimportant. On the contrary, Newell (1999) has noted that Price's model remains of interest for four reasons at least. First, it is one of very few such models to go beyond simple statement of the distinction between perceptual and evaluative aspects of body image. Any model which recognises the complexity of body image and attempts to codify it in a meaningful way is important. Second, the model has a high profile amongst British nurses at a time when comparatively little emphasis is placed on body image outside the field of eating disorders. Third, it is explicitly tied to clinical practice, from whose observations it is drawn and to which its implications are linked in the form of recommendations for nursing activity. Academic activity which links to practice is to be applauded. Finally, it has been influential in increasing nurses' awareness of body image issues and stimulating debate. In spite of these strengths, however, because of the shortcomings outlined above, Price's model of body image remains a set of untested assumptions and is, in consequence, purely speculative (Gournay *et al.* 1997).

An important further account of body image disturbance and adaptation from the nursing literature is suggested by Dropkin (1989). Her model draws considerably on Lazarus's (1966) formulations of stress and coping, and is also related to Lang's (1971) three systems model. Dropkin's model was developed principally in the context of postoperative recovery following head and neck surgery for cancer. According to Dropkin, the surgical procedure for removal of cancer is seen, in Lazarus's terms, as the *stressor* to which adaptation is required. The person's cognitive appraisal of this threat leads to a series of affective and physiological responses which interact with behavioural responses. These behavioural responses are seen as indicative of adaptation, or what Dropkin describes as body image reintegration, when they involve 'confrontation, compliance and redefinition'. Confrontation may be both behavioural and cognitive, whilst compliance is chiefly concerned with following the instructions of clinicians, particularly as these relate to self-care and confrontation. The redefinition element of her model involves a changing of the person's value system following disfiguring surgery towards an appreciation that change in appearance or function does not change the nature of the person. Self-care, grooming and socialisation are viewed as key elements of this process. Dropkin has extensively investigated the postoperative behaviours of head and neck patients, using this stress-coping model (Scott *et al.* 1980), and reported the need for the performance of self-care tasks, including socialisation tasks, during the first eight postoperative days (Dropkin and Scott 1983). Dropkin (1989) suggests that these tasks, when successfully completed, are associated with adaptation and reintegration.

From the viewpoint of the cognitive-behavioural approach to be introduced in this study, Dropkin's approach has considerable attraction. As noted above, it shares a similar general view of human behaviour and experience with the three systems model often practised in cognitive-behaviour therapy. More critically, it emphasises the importance of behavioural confrontation and, to a lesser extent, attitude change. The first of these, in particular, is seen as important in cognitive-behavioural approaches, described in more detail later in this book. However, Dropkin's approach has a number of shortcomings. First, her investigations are almost exclusively in the field of cancer surgery, where the patient may have to adapt to many stressors other than those involving disfigurement (e.g. loss of function, receiving a diagnosis of a life-threatening disease, the necessity to change lifestyle radically, persistent fear of recurrence). This is a potential source of difficulty for her model since many of the experiences noted in her patients may have more to do with adaptation to these threats than adaptation to threats to body image. Since, in her study groups, the possible interactions between issues of body image, physical illness and diagnosis are not adequately controlled, we may be seeing, in Dropkin's work, a model of adaptation to life-threatening illness in general. That these issues need isolating is not in doubt, since in a recent study (Newell 2000) it was found that people who had undergone plastic surgery for cancer were significantly *less* psychologically disturbed than those who had had such surgery for revision of scarring from other sources. Likewise, the responses Dropkin and Scott (1983) observe as a result of interventions may also be peculiar to recovery after cancer.

As a second potential drawback, Dropkin is concerned primarily with short-term adjustment during the postoperative period. This is an extremely important area, but is once again a potential source of contamination by issues of threat to the self other than those to body image, such as fear, pain, disability. Third, although the role of self-care tasks and socialisation is explained in terms of Lazarus's model, the precise process by which completion of such tasks leads to adaptation is not described. More importantly, despite considerable close descriptive examination of the performance of such tasks by patients, no adequate investigation of cause and effect relationships between these tasks and psychosocial adjustment exists. Despite these difficulties, Dropkin's work has been an important influence upon the model to be presented in this book, principally because of the emphasis in her work on confrontation and its supposed effect on successful adjustment.

A considerable amount of interest in body image has been generated by the clinical needs of those involved in treatment of its disturbances, in particular the eating disorders. From a cognitive-behavioural perspective, Slade (1994), who has written extensively about eating disorders, describes an account of body image development and disturbance which has considerable concordance with the cognitive-behavioural approach which underpins this book. The organisation of the components of the model is very similar to an earlier fear and avoidance model of pain perception in whose formulation Slade participated (Lethem et al. 1983; Slade et al. 1983). In outlining his approach, Slade (1994) notes the convergence of approaches from observations of perceptual defects in neurological disorders, the body image distortion in eating and weight disorders and the 'delusional misperception' of body dysmorphic disorder (BDD). In BDD, the sufferer believes that some bodily feature or function is offensive to others. According to Slade, the genesis of approaches to body image in these three clinical fields has led to a notion that body image disorder is primarily perceptual in nature. Slade also argues, on the other hand, that not only is this a mistaken emphasis, but that even the apparent measurement of perceptual phenomena involves people in judgements which owe a great deal to issues such as attitude, affect and cognition.

Much of the rationale for Slade's emphasis on these components of body image rather than perceptual aspects is derived from work with eating disorders and relates to interventions with these conditions. A detailed discussion of these elements of his work is beyond the scope of this book. He draws the following general conclusions regarding body image. The mental representation of the body is not fixed but fluctuates within a limited range (the body image band). In the absence of emotional and attitudinal biases, estimates of that representation will be in the middle of the band. By contrast, strong concern about, for example, body size will result in judgements of size at the limits of the range. Thus, perceptual awareness or judgement of size in eating disorders are affected by pre-existing and shifting emotional and attitudinal biases. Previously, commentators such as Bruch (1962) had characterised anorexia nervosa sufferers as possessing a fixed distorted body image of delusional proportions, and this characteristic has been widely regarded as a defining feature of the disorder, but Slade suggests, by contrast, that sufferers possess an uncertain, unstable and weak body image. This, he suggests, is translated into overly cautious perceptual estimates. This view might possibly be extended to apply to BDD sufferers who, it might be suggested, have a similarly unstable image of a particular bodily attribute or function which is likewise overemphasised in situations of stress such as social interaction.

The general model of body image development which Slade (1994) has constructed consists of the following seven components, all of which influence what he describes as the 'loose mental representation of the body' he says best describes body image. A history of sensory input to the body regarding its form, size, shape and appearance gives a general mental representation of the body. Cultural and social norms about the body inform both attitudes to weight and shape and the general body image, whilst individual attitudes both input directly to body image and affect cognitive and affective variables. Biological variables also impact on body image. In the context of eating disorders, one such factor might be basal metabolic rate. The final two elements of Slade's model are both particular to disorders of body image. Individual psychopathology such as anorexia nervosa both influences body image and is influenced by factors such as cultural norms and cognitive and affective variables, whilst, in eating disorders, a history of weight change is construed as leading to a broadening of the body image band, and thus a loosening of the body image. The arrangement of the various elements is shown in Figure 2.2.

Like Price's (1990a, 1990b) model, Slade's view of body image has not been empirically tested. However, confidence in its usefulness as a way of examining body image may be strengthened by two factors. Slade has drawn on empirical evidence from both clinical and experimental studies of eating disorders in the construction of the model, and the use of such well-constructed studies in support of a model is a useful advance on simply speculative accounts. Moreover, his model is closely related to an earlier fear and avoidance model of pain perception (Lethem *et al.* 1983; Slade *et al.* 1983) which has proved of some use in predicting results in the examination of pain in clinical settings (Rose *et al.* 1992). This predictive value, if it proves robust in the context of body image disturbance, is likely to prove important, since it will help to establish the validity of Slade's approach as a guide to intervention.

Unlike Price's approach, Slade's (1994) model is narrow in focus in two senses. It is essentially a model of bodily perception, in which attitudes and other elements of appraisal or satisfaction with the body

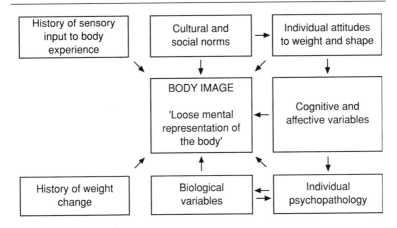

Figure 2.2 Slade's model of body image disturbance (after Slade 1994)

play a secondary part, being contributing factors to the development of the representation of the body. Whilst a 'loose mental representation of the body' appears a sufficiently broad term to include attitudinal and affective elements of body image, it is clear from the general context of Slade's paper that his model is one with inputs and outputs, in which attitudinal aspects do not feature as outputs. Moreover, the main focus of his model is upon perception in general and size in particular.

The second limitation of his approach concerns the patient group from which it is derived. Since the model is based on an examination of the pathology of eating disorders, from which all the supporting examples are drawn, extrapolations to other disorders of body image must be made with caution. Generalising to body image in a well population is even more problematic. Whilst Price's model is perhaps too broad in focus, Slade's seems to be too narrow to be of general applicability without modification.

Nevertheless, such modification need not be drastic. Exchanging *individual psychopathology* for *personality variables* as in the Lethem *et al.* (1983) model of pain perception (see Chapter 3) and changing *history of weight change* to *history of bodily changes* together serve to illustrate how the model might be applied more broadly to body image disturbance, such as disfigurement. With this greater generalisability, the model might be appropriately extended to include well populations. Moreover, it is not necessary to retain Slade's (1994) emphasis on the perceptual element of representation. Indeed, since one of the aims of his paper is to demonstrate how perceptual judgements are influenced by such factors as attitude and affect, it is a small step to speculate on how the various inputs in Slade's model might lead to differences in attitudes to the body. For example, Newell's (1991) discussion of how reinforcement might account for the development of aspects of attitudes to the body may easily be applied to an examination of the ways in which cultural and social norms might lead to alterations in both the perceptual and *attitudinal* aspects of body image. The same is true of Slade's own discussion of how elements within his own model contribute to perceptual changes. In consequence, there is no need for us to assume that the perceptual element has any primacy in the resulting 'loose mental representation'. Thus, the seven elements of Slade's (1994) general model of body image may be construed as contributing equally to a body image which is both perceptual and 'attitudinal, affective and cognitive' (Slade 1988).

Approaches to measurement of body image

Measurement of body image has moved from earlier, more general approaches towards multidimensional measures of body image, and we now turn to an examination of this trend. For the moment, we will look at measurement in quite a general way, returning in later chapters to mention highly specific measurement tactics in experimental and clinical studies when we examine the studies themselves. It should be noted, however, that clinical practice has suffered from a lack of generally used, valid measures of body image, certainly outside the field of mental health care. Even here, measurement of this kind has generally been restricted to the eating disorders.

Measurement of body image has generally reflected the division between perceptual and attitudinal/affective components described earlier in this chapter. A review of measurement techniques by McCrea *et al.* (1982), dealing mainly with measurement of body perception, concluded that the great breadth of sources from which investigation of body image has occurred has led to a tendency towards vague, equivocal definitions of the concept. Moreover, this vagueness has itself led to a proliferation of measurement approaches, which has become a handicap within the field. However, this issue has mainly affected judgement of perception rather than attitude. The measurement of attitude has received rather more attention, although once again the coverage of the field has been sketchy. This book is primarily concerned with evaluative aspects of body image – the thoughts, feelings and behaviours which attach to or comprise one's attitudes to one's body. As a consequence, this part will deal only with the measurement of these evaluative aspects of body image, rather than the individual's ability to perceive the body's shape and size.

Secord (1953) constructed the earliest systematised scale to examine elements of body image. The original purpose of this work was only loosely involved with body image, but had a more theoretical aim. It was designed as a modification of Jung's word association methods to allow this technique to be used in a reliable way across groups of subjects, rather than the ideographic approach of Jung's earlier work. Words possibly associated with the body were merely the stimulus materials. Seventy-five homonyms with either body or non-body meanings (e.g. colon = gut *or* punctuation mark) were presented to subjects. There are considerable difficulties with the lack of specificity of the language of the paper, which reflects the analytical tradition from which it springs and need not concern us here, since they relate to the possible clinical relevance of the measure within that tradition. From the point of view of the study of body image, the important element of the study was that it demonstrated that people thought to have different personality structures reliably interpreted the homonyms in different ways (either as body-related or not). The study was, therefore, an early attempt to systematise examination of attitudes to the body.

More importantly, the scale devised for the study was the forerunner of the Body Cathexis Scale (Secord and Jourard 1953) which overcame many of the methodological and interpretational difficulties of its predecessor and became a widely used tool in the investigation of body image.

The Body Cathexis Scale investigates only *cathexis* (the level of an individual's feeling of satisfaction or dissatisfaction with bodily parts or processes) and consists of five-point scales related to 46 body parts or functions, indicating different levels of satisfaction. The authors hypothesised that bodily feelings would be similar to feelings about the self and that negative feelings about the body would be associated with anxiety and with negative feelings about the self. Thus, a second part of the scale contained fifty-five items related to aspects of the self.

Moderately strong correlations were found between the body cathexis and self cathexis elements (0.58 for men and 0.66 for women), indicating a correspondence between satisfaction with the body and with the self. This finding adds weight to the assertion of a relationship between body image and self image in Price (1990a) and the Freudian notion that the ego is predominantly an expression of the body (Bronheim *et al.* 1991), but it must be noted that the level of these correlations still indicates considerable *divergence between* attitudes to one's body and one's self.

The self and the body are clearly linked, but the relationship between them requires much further investigation. In a later study (Jourard and Secord 1954) body cathexis was found to be moderately but significantly related to many aspects of body size (height, shoulder width, chest, biceps, muscular strength) in sixty-two male undergraduates.

Bruchon-Schweitzer (1987) notes that although it has remained the most frequently used such measure, the Body Cathexis Scale measures only one dimension of body image: satisfaction. This is not quite accurate, since elements of the scale have been used as proxy measures of anxiety (Secord and Jourard 1953), but it is true that this latter aspect of the scale has received considerably less attention than the more general concept of bodily satisfaction. Bruchon-Schweitzer (1987) suggested that body image was multidimensional and derived a body image questionnaire of 19 items from interviews with 137 high school students. This questionnaire was then administered to 619 subjects and the results factor analysed in order to establish construct validity. Four stable factors were found: accessibility/closeness; satisfaction/dissatisfaction; activity/ passivity; relaxation/tension. The identification of these component factors of body image enables investigators to move away from a global examination of the phenomenon towards more precise specification both of elements of body image and of their possible relationships with other variables. For example, the Bruchon-Schweitzer study found a positive correlation between body satisfaction and extroversion on the Eysenck Personality Inventory (EPI) and negative correlations between body activity and relaxation and EPI neuroticism scales. Although the identification of such possible dimensions is potentially important, as a means of examining body image and its disturbance with greater focus and sensitivity, it should also be noted that the Bruchon-Schweitzer (1987) questionnaire (the Body Image Questionnaire) has not found its way into general use in *clinical* literature in the field of body image disturbance, and its use has not been reported in nursing.

The multidimensional nature of body image has also been explored by Cash (1989) and Brown *et al.* (1990). Cash *et al.*'s (1986) Body Self Relations Questionnaire (BSRQ) was designed to take into account cognitive and behavioural factors as well as the affect examined by the Body Cathexis Scale, in order to reflect more accurately the concept of an *attitude*, which should contain these diverse elements of experience. The scale consists of fifty-four items and was tested on 2052 subjects and factor analysed to yield seven factors: appearance evaluation, appearance orientation, fitness evaluation, fitness orientation, health evaluation, health orientation and illness orientation, which were consistent across the sexes. The authors concluded that their findings supported the existence of separate dimensions of body image experience and that investigators should both beware of the 'uniformity myth' of the body image construct and distinguish between perceptual and attitudinal modalities. Although Cash, who originated the scale, has worked a great deal in the field of body image *disorder* and anorexia nervosa, the scale's norms were established on general population samples (Cash *et al.* 1986) and the Brown *et al.* (1990) study likewise used such normal subjects, in this case stratified to represent the sex and age distribution of the US population. As a result of this careful use of a subject group to identify the elements of the scale, their conclusions regarding dimensions of body image are likewise based upon the general population rather than clinical population subjects, adding to the scale's generalisability. As a consequence, we may feel that the scale's applicability for clinical practice is similarly widened. It is also worth contrasting the empirical basis for the different elements of body image they assert with the speculative approach of Price (1990a, 1990b) and, to a lesser extent, Slade (1994).

The Cash (1989) paper further adds to our understanding of the multidimensional nature of body image by demonstrating that, whilst assessment of body image attitudes may be divided into examination of the whole body and of individual body parts, the individual elements do not contribute *equally* to overall evaluation of the body. Specifically, Cash found that weight, upper torso, face, mid torso, lower torso and muscle tone (in descending order of importance) predicted overall appearance satisfaction and self-rated attractiveness in men, with only height satisfaction making no predictive contribution. In women, weight, upper torso, mid torso, lower torso and face predicted the general measures, with height and muscle tone making no contribution. Cash concluded that body part and global satisfaction converge, and that most body parts make a unique and additive contribution to the general appraisal of the body, but these contributions are not equal. The opportunity to use the BSRQ to assess body image and its disturbance in clinical practice is potentially exciting, particularly given the possibility of isolating attitudes to different parts of the body. However, despite the broad population base employed in its validation, its clinical use has largely remained restricted to mental health settings.

Summary

Body image is generally divided into the consideration of ~~~ceptual and evaluative aspects, and much of the study of these elements is derived from an examination of their disturbance, particularly from the field of eating disorders. Major drawbacks of current models of body image include lack of empirical testing of the models and lack of predictive value; inadequate description of the way elements of the models are related; lack of comprehensivity in the areas of body image addressed; and a focus on disturbance rather than normal body image.

Measurement of body image reflects the distinction between perceptual and attitudinal/affective elements, although only the latter are examined in this book. The works of Secord and his collaborators and, much more recently, Cash and his collaborators provide us with a means of investigating normal body image, in order to give a source of information against which to examine its disturbances. Some opportunity is available to isolate attitudes to specific body parts. These measures are not extensively used in clinical practice.

Exercise

Consider a key threat to one's body image. Ideally, this will be something you have experienced yourself. If not, perhaps you have a friend or relative who has faced such a threat. This may be as a result of illness or injury, or may be developmental.

How did you/they address these difficulties? Consider this under these headings:

- What did you feel physically?
- What were your emotions?
- What were your key thoughts?
- How did you behave?

Now consider how these activities affected your reactions to the threat you have focused upon.

Key further reading

Dropkin, M.J. and Scott, D.W. (1983) Body image reintegration and coping effectiveness after head and neck surgery. *Journal of Social Otorhinolaryngological Head and Neck Nursing* 2, 7–16.

An important investigation of how people might come to terms with altered body image in the context of a life-threatening illness.

Newell, R. (1991) Body image disturbance: cognitive-behavioural formulation and intervention. *Journal of Advanced Nursing* 16, 1400–5.

An earlier formulation of the model of body image described in this book, but focusing chiefly on disturbance rather than normal body image.

Price, R. (1990b) *Body Image: Nursing Concepts and Care*. New York: Prentice-Hall.

The most influential UK nursing writer on body image matters.

Schilder, P. (1935) *Image and Appearance of the Human Body*. London: Kegan Paul.

The classic early text describing body image in health and illness.

Chapter 3

The cognitive-behavioural approach to body image and its disturbance

Behavioural and cognitive approaches to human distress

In Chapter 2, a number of general approaches to body image and its measurement were described, and it was noted that there are shortcomings with current models of body image and its disturbance. This chapter introduces a model of body image and its disturbance, the fear–avoidance model, which attempts to address some of these difficulties. In particular, the model aims to be relatively comprehensive in the aspects of body image and its disturbance which it addresses, and to allow us to test its usefulness through empirical studies of the assertions it makes. The model is firmly grounded in a broader cognitive-behavioural approach to human experience, and in behavioural and cognitive therapies for human distress. These approaches have themselves been subjected to prolonged and rigorous evaluation, most recently in major reviews of treatment studies (Fonagy and Roth 1996; Department of Health 1999). This evaluation continues as the effective elements of treatment are further isolated and as the approach is applied to other areas of human distress. A full review of the literature which addresses the effectiveness of the cognitive-behavioural (CB) approach is beyond the scope of this book, but the opening sections of this chapter examine the CB approach in general terms, in order to introduce the reader to the basis for the CB approach to body image, its disturbance and psychological difficulties in disfigurement.

We will examine the potential contribution of cognitive-behaviour therapy (CBT) to the understanding and treatment of psychological consequences of disfigurement. As will be seen in later chapters, none of the intervention studies with such psychological disturbances have specifically defined their theoretical underpinnings in cognitive-behavioural terms. Similarly, there has been no specifically cognitive-behavioural formulation stated in the literature for the genesis and maintenance of these difficulties other than Newell (1991, 1999). However, cognitive-behaviour therapy approaches to a number of other psychological problems offer potential insights into the difficulties of disfigured people. The development of the CBT approach from its roots in behaviour therapy will be traced, and the main treatment techniques used to address focal anxieties such as phobias will be described. A brief synoptic account will be given of the empirical status of these techniques, and the case of social phobia will be considered in more detail, principally because of its relevance to disfigured people and their social difficulties (Newell and Marks 2000).

Development of behaviour therapy

Modern behaviour therapy consists of a number of elements which are typically derived from learning theories, especially those concerned with operant and classical conditioning, and, more recently, with social learning theories (Newell 1996). Strict behaviourists argue that internal motivating processes such as thoughts and feelings are both opaque to the client and therapist and possibly irrelevant to the process or outcome of therapy. Although agreement with such assertions varies amongst therapists, they are generally united in their belief that client *behaviour* is the most important aetiological and maintaining factor in client difficulties. Individual client problems are seen as instances of inappropriate learning, with treatment seeking either to undo the effects of such learning or to initiate new learnt behaviours incompatible with problematic aspects of the client's life.

Problem behaviours are always the direct focus of treatment, and little discussion of underlying causes will take place (Marks 1986). Most behaviour therapists minimise or deny the importance of such assumed causes, and some assert that the notions of cause and symptom are inappropriate applications of medical models to psychological distress. Medical practitioners tend to think in terms of symptoms being indicative of certain causal pathogens. Treating only symptoms is regarded as inappropriate because the causal agent, if unaddressed, will simply cause the symptoms to recur. This notion of symptom and cause was applied by early psychotherapists, in all probability because of their medical background. Thus, it was felt that clients' psychological difficulties were 'symptoms' of some underlying psychological 'cause' in a way similar to physical illness. By contrast, behavioural theorists argue that all human behaviour is either innate or the result of learning. This is as true of maladaptive behaviours as of adaptive ones. We do not describe *adaptive* behaviours as symptomatic of some underlying pathology, so there is no logical reason to do so with problem behaviours (Newell 1996).

Behaviour therapy is a wide-ranging approach, and has been applied to many different client difficulties, from anxiety-based disorders, to education of people with learning disabilities, to behavioural medicine. In our examination of the difficulties arising from disturbed body image, we will be chiefly concerned with anxiety and its treatment. Arguably the most significant therapeutic advance in the treatment of phobic anxiety was the notion of 'reciprocal inhibition', developed by Joseph Wolpe (1958). Wolpe was originally trained in psychoanalysis, but came to be critical of the apparent lack of ability of this therapy to alleviate the problems of clients. He derived the concept of reciprocal inhibition from observations, during animal work on induced fear, that feeding behaviour was inhibited during induction of the fear response. He hypothesised that anxiety might therefore be inhibited by feeding, and that such inhibition of anxiety, if demonstrated, might prove useful in clinical treatment of neurotic complaints (Wolpe 1952).

Wolpe extended his animal work to address the difficulties of human clients, typically using relaxation (Wolpe 1958) as the response said to 'reciprocally inhibit' anxiety. In psychotherapy by reciprocal inhibition, the client visualised a hierarchy of situations which successively approximate to the feared situation, relaxing at each stage. When each situation could be visualised without anxiety, the client progressed to the next. Finally, the situations were confronted in real life. This form of 'systematic desensitisation' has an excellent success rate with many anxiety-based disorders (Rachman and Wilson 1980), and has been demonstrated to have outcomes superior to traditional verbal psychotherapies, even in reviews conducted by commentators sympathetic to such psychoanalytically oriented treatments (Smith and Glass 1977). It also appears that treatments based upon reciprocal inhibition are as effective as more modern cognitively led interventions (see later in this chapter).

Reciprocal inhibition is said to operate principally by the mechanism of extinction, whereby an organism ceases to demonstrate a conditioned response (fear) to a conditioned stimulus (say, a large store in the case of an agoraphobic) when it is presented in the absence of its associated unconditioned stimulus (e.g. autonomic arousal). By contrast, flooding, and the more recent exposure therapies (Marks 1987), are described as operating principally as a consequence of habituation, that most basic process of learning, whereby an organism ceases to respond to a repeatedly presented stimulus (Walker 1987). Thus, in exposure, the individual is confronted, typically in real life rather than in imagination, by the feared situation, and encouraged to remain there until such time as anxiety subsides as a consequence of habituation. It has been demonstrated that the results of this approach are, in phobias, at least as effective as reciprocal inhibition. Moreover, the approach avoids the necessity to teach relaxation exercises or to construct complicated hierarchies, with resulting saving in time for both client and therapist. Exposure instructions can be offered both by a human therapist and by the use of proxies such as computer programs and self-help manuals (Marks 1987).

The dominant theoretical model of the acquisition and maintenance of problematic behaviours was, for a considerable time, the two factor (Mowrer 1960) or two process theory (Gray 1975), which asserted that problems such as phobias arose as a result of classical conditioning, but were maintained by operant conditioning, principally through the mechanism of negative reinforcement. Thus, the agoraphobic in the example above *acquires* the fear of shopping in a large store by pairing the unconditioned stimulus of, for example, the chance occurrence of untoward bodily symptoms (perhaps a consequence of some minor physical illness) with the conditioned stimulus of the surroundings of the store, which in turn comes to elicit a conditioned response of subjective feelings of anxiety, even in the absence of the original eliciting bodily symptoms. This response is repeated in similar situations through the process of generalisation, in which organisms respond to stimuli similar to the one to which their conditioned response has been trained (Walker 1984). However, the agoraphobic response is generally *maintained* by active and passive avoidance. When in the feared situation, the client experiences the aversive physical sensations of anxiety, and rapidly leaves the situation. This leads to a diminution in the aversive sensations, a situation which, according to the operant principle of negative reinforcement, increases the likelihood of future instances of the behaviour which has led to this diminution, in this case, escape behaviour.

Whilst exposure theory relies principally on the notion of habituation, it can be seen that the action of remaining in the feared situation until anxiety has subsided also stops the reinforcement of escape behaviour, because the client experiences anxiety reduction not as a result of escape, but as a result of remaining in the situation and allowing habituation to occur. Since escape behaviour is no longer reinforced, its frequency reduces.

Social learning

Behaviour therapy has been historically an eclectic tradition, drawing on numerous elements of learning theory. The social learning theory of Albert Bandura (1977a) was incorporated into behaviour therapy practice at a relatively early date and marks a progression from behaviour therapy to cognitive-behaviour therapy. Both social learning theory and the therapeutic use of modelling (the process whereby individuals tend to imitate behaviours which they have observed being reinforced in others) have a clear basis in operant conditioning. However, social learning implies considerable *cognitive* processing by the client, whose own behaviour is not itself *directly* reinforced. The client thus has to construct, through observation, an expectation of reinforcement. Bandura's work both recognises the existence of such processes and describes them as influencing the surrounding environment as well as being influenced by it. Social learning theory is thus less deterministic than operant and classical learning theories. Bandura has developed treatment interventions based on social learning theory and modelling, involving acquisition of desired behaviours such as social skills or approach to feared situations following demonstration and reinforcement of these skills by the therapist or some other appropriate model. This modelling may also be carried out via cognitive rehearsal of desired behaviours, symbolic modelling through writing and speaking, or the processes of self-monitoring, self-modelling and self-reinforcement (Bandura 1986). The link between the work of Bandura and that of the cognitive theorists, and of cognitive and cognitive-behaviour therapists, lies in his acknowledgement of the importance of internal processes in determining behaviour.

Behaviour therapy and cognitive therapy

Behaviour therapy and behavioural accounts of human experiences have been criticised on a number of grounds. Behaviour therapy is by no means universally effective, even where it is the treatment of choice. There are numerous conditions which, whilst causing significant distress, contain little, if any, observable behaviour upon which treatment can focus. Insufficient detail is said to be paid by behaviour therapy to the client–therapist relationship and adherence to therapeutic instructions (Hawton *et al.* 1989). Each of these arguments is capable of refutation (Newell and Dryden 1991). Although few would argue that behaviourism (or indeed any other account) is a complete description of human experience, the imperfection of behaviour therapy as a treatment is not necessarily an indication of this lack of completeness, but could equally be caused by such issues as inadequate assessment of the problem, therapist inexperience or lack of adherence to clinical instructions by the client. Similarly, the lack of emphasis upon the therapeutic relationship is a criticism not of the theory of behaviour therapy itself, but of the way in which it may sometimes be practised, and, indeed, behaviourists have expended a good deal of energy in attempting to understand this relationship, particularly as it bears on adherence. The most that can be said is that behaviour therapy does not primarily *use* the relationship as the mechanism by which treatment is expected to work. Finally, whilst lack of observable behaviour has in the past represented both a therapeutic and a theoretical problem for behaviour therapists, some disorders without such behaviour have nevertheless been successfully addressed, most notably obsessional thoughts (Salkovskis and Kirk 1989). Moreover, some behaviourists explicitly admit the existence of and work with cognitive processes, but simply assert that these processes are subject to the same laws of conditioning as overt behaviours (Jaremko 1986). Nevertheless, for many researchers and therapists, strictly behavioural accounts of human distress have come to be regarded as too simple to account for the complexity of many everyday human behaviours, such as speech.

Cognitive therapy consists of a broad range of accounts of the genesis and maintenance of human difficulties and of their treatment. For example, Rachman and Wilson (1980) noted that the founders of two dominant forces, Beck's cognitive therapy (1976) and Ellis's rational–emotive therapy (1962), had their professional beginnings in psychoanalysis, whilst Meichenbaum (1977), who developed self-instructional training and cognitive-behaviour modification, came from the behavioural tradition. Their therapies reflect some of this difference in origins, but are united to a considerable degree by their development principally from clinical situations and observations. By contrast, later accounts have attempted to integrate such observations with developments in cognitive psychology, using computer analogues of human information processing and empirical studies of the cognitive processes of non-clinical populations (Newell and Dryden 1991). Nevertheless, these varying approaches share at least four key similarities. They all agree that thoughts exist, mediate client problems, are capable of change by therapist and client and are the primary focus of therapeutic endeavours towards such change (Newell and Dryden 1991).

The cognitive therapies stress the importance of a mediating, or even causative, role for cognitions. Beck's (1967) description of the 'cognitive triad' of negative thoughts about the self, the world and the future as the key feature of depression is now widely accepted, both in cognitive therapy and in mainstream psychiatry, whilst his notion of 'modes' of thinking offers a rationale for the development of different client problems. Thus, if an individual is overactive in terms of an anxious mode of thinking, this might both activate anxiety schema in the presence of relatively trivial threats and lead to continuing activity of these schema after the threat has passed (Beck and Emery 1985). This conceptualisation of anxiety is, like much of the work of Beck and Ellis, based primarily on observation of clinical populations, and owes comparatively little to cognitive psychology, although later cognitive therapists and researchers have attempted to account for these notions by reference to mainstream cognitive psychology and its associated research methods. Whilst there is evidence that the cognitive therapies of Beck and Ellis are effective, at least in depression, this success may owe as much to pragmatic elements of the therapy as to the purported theories of cognition embodied in them. However, some studies do suggest the existence of cognitive biases such as those suggested by cognitive therapists. For example, an early study by Bradley and Mathews (1988) found depressed subjects recalled more negative material referring to the self than did either recovering depressed clients or controls, whilst the recovering depressives recalled more negative material related to others. For cognitive therapy, this study is important in two ways. First, it supports the existence of two aspects of Beck's cognitive triad (negative thoughts about the self and others) in depressed and recovering depressed individuals and, more importantly, it suggests, in the finding for recovering depressed individuals, the existence of some mediating element in this response bias which is more enduring than a simple effect of mood. A Beckian 'schema' could represent such an element. The Bradley and Mathews (1988) experiment represents one of a number of attempts to investigate the assumptions of cognitive therapy using the methods and theoretical constructs of academic cognitive psychology. These attempts are reviewed by Brewin (1988).

In brief, behaviour therapy may be characterised as a concentration on modification of the effects of faulty *conditioning*, whilst cognitive therapy may be summarised as a concentration on addressing the effects of faulty *thinking*. Thus cognitive therapists educate clients as to this model for their difficulties and train them to recognise, monitor and challenge such dysfunctional thinking when it occurs. Since cognitive therapists regard errors in thinking as causative of client difficulties such as depression and anxiety, the modification of such errors in thinking is believed to lead to improvement. However, criticism of cognitive therapy has arisen from a variety of sources. Wolpe has been extremely sceptical of the claims of cognitive therapy in treatment of anxiety, and questioned its distinctiveness as a form of intervention (Wolpe 1978), whilst Marks (1987) has noted that many of the supposed effects of cognitive therapy could be accounted for by a simpler mechanism, such as habituation. Furthermore, cognitive therapies have always included elements of behavioural experimentation (aimed at testing faulty cognitions), increasing the likelihood that such mechanisms as anxiety reduction through habituation, rather than restructuring of dysfunctional cognitions, might be responsible for improvement. A number of studies have attempted to dismantle the differing elements of treatment, but this is not always easy, because of the insistence of cognitive therapy on the use of behavioural experimentation. However, a meta-analysis of studies examining cognitive therapy with a range of anxiety-based disorders (Berman *et al.* 1985) found no difference between cognitive therapy, systematic desensitisation and a combination of these treatments. The analysis was well conducted, taking reasonable care to include well-constructed studies. It differed from an earlier analysis by Shapiro and Shapiro (1982) which found an advantage for cognitive therapy. Most recently, a well-conducted meta-analysis by Taylor (1996) showed superiority of a range of cognitive-behavioural interventions over placebo, with a combination of cognitive therapy and exposure performing most reliably, whilst another recent review (Stavynski and Greenberg 1998) showed that results of the range of cognitive-behavioural interventions resulted in long-lasting improvement. Neither study, however, provides conclusive evidence for any major contribution of cognitive therapy in the absence of behavioural elements.

Cognitive-behaviour therapy

Whilst cognitive therapy has been characterised as emphasising the primacy of cognitions in determining client difficulties and behaviour therapy as stressing the primacy of behaviours, cognitive-behavioural approaches take both a more varied view of causation and a more pragmatic approach to therapy. These approaches certainly retain an emphasis on cognition, but are likely to examine other response systems when arriving at a formulation of the origins and maintenance of particular client difficulties. A relatively durable approach to the assessment and treatment of client difficulties is the three systems model advocated by Lang (1971) and later refined by Rachman and Hodgson (1974). Lang (1971) divided human experience and client problems into three systems:

physiological activity (in particular, in the context of anxiety, autonomic activity), behaviour, and cognitive activity (as revealed by verbal report). Intervention by the therapist might be directed at whichever of the systems appeared primarily affected, employing a primarily physiologically, behaviourally or cognitively oriented set of interventions, such as relaxation, exposure, or cognitive restructuring respectively. It is this flexibility and willingness to embrace differing techniques which distinguishes cognitive-behavioural approaches from more traditional behaviour therapy or cognitive therapy. However, it is worth repeating that cognitive therapy had contained behavioural elements since its inception, whilst cognitive aspects of experience were integrated into behaviour at a very early stage, through the use of, for example, modelling, teaching new skills, and self-monitoring. This suggests that differences between the practice of cognitive and behaviour therapy may have been less than an examination of their theoretical standpoints would lead the observer to expect. Indeed, the Berman *et al.* (1985) review mentioned above found considerable overlap in terms of the procedures employed by the two orientations. It has been suggested that, rather than speaking of a distinct cognitive-behaviour therapy, it may be more appropriate to refer to cognitive-behavioural orientations (Newell and Dryden 1991). Such orientations will lead to treatment interventions which take account of cognitive elements of human experience to varying degrees.

Behaviour therapy and cognitive-behaviour therapy today are generally eclectic approaches (Newell 1996), in which the therapist chooses from a range of techniques which have generally been empirically tested and received some level of support. In examining unfamiliar client difficulties, the therapist attempts to proceed in a way which draws on these techniques and applies them in unfamiliar circumstances whilst attempting to construct treatment in an experimental way which allows both client and therapist to assess the effectiveness of the interventions used. Both the use of empirically tested treatment methods and the continuing use of scientific method to test new treatment approaches have been continuing themes which have lasted from the inception of behaviour therapy in the middle of this century until the present day, when cognitive-behaviour therapy represents the most widely investigated and supported mode of intervention for a wide range of client difficulties (Rachman and Wilson 1980; Fonagy and Roth 1996). As with nursing, behaviour therapy and its variants face a continuing challenge to ensure that clinically effective practices gain acceptance amongst practitioners whilst approaches which have the support of clinicians from their often biased experiences fade from their therapeutic repertoires. Debate over both theory and clinical efficacy have been part of behaviour therapy and its successors since its inception, and it is important to recognise that the therapeutic orientation of behaviourism is sufficiently concerned with scientific rigour to allow such debate to continue.

Cognitive-behaviour therapy and social phobia

Phobic disorders in general are characterised by irrational fear and avoidance of particular objects or situations. It has been suggested by Seligman (1971) that phobias, although learned and maintained through the processes of classical and operant conditioning, are also genetically prepared. The phenomenon of preparedness leads humans to be more likely to develop phobias towards entities or situations which are potentially dangerous to the species. Thus, such phobias as fear of heights, enclosed spaces, certain animals, are likely to occur commonly because fear and avoidance of these things has a potential survival value for our species.

The case of social phobia is more complex, since fear of social situations is most often coupled with fear of some more abstract entity such as negative appraisal or ostracism by others (Butler 1989). Sufferers typically avoid social situations, and this may be highly specific, being confined, for example, to eating with others, being in group situations or dating, or may extend to a broad range of social situations. The sufferer may fear negative appraisal, rejection, inability to perform, panic or even collapse, and the complaint is often accompanied by severe situational autonomic arousal (Butler 1989). However, fear of negative appraisal in social situations may indeed have survival value. The human species is highly social, and isolation from others as a result of their negative appraisal has obvious negative consequences with regard to the survival of both an individual and her/his genetic material. Individuals who are negatively appraised might be deprived of the support of the group in times of hardship and less likely to mate. Thus there may be good reason to speculate that fear of negative social appraisal is genetically prepared. Unfortunately, the avoidance behaviours associated with this fear lack survival value, since they are themselves associated with isolation.

Cognitive-behaviour therapy is the treatment of choice for social phobia and typically contains major components of exposure to the feared situations. In a recent review of CBT approaches to anxiety, Chambless and Gillis (1993) conclude that CBT has consistently demonstrated results superior to waiting list and placebo controls and to supportive psychotherapy. However, the addition of specifically cognitive elements did not unequivocally appear to contribute to treatment effectiveness, with only two out of eight comparative studies resulting in greater improvement with such additions. One of these studies (Butler *et al.* 1984) was particularly well carried out, using a demonstrably credible ineffective 'filler' treatment to control for the extra time involved in adding group anxiety management to exposure treatment. The addition of anxiety management appeared to lead to greater resilience against relapse. Differences between exposure alone and exposure plus anxiety management were apparent on more measures at follow-up than post treatment, and considerably more exposure patients sought further treatment during the follow-up. However, the numbers in the study were small (15 per group) and a replication of this study would be welcome, particularly since Chambless and Gillis (1993) alert us to the dangers of introducing combination treatments without good evidence.

Towards a cognitive-behavioural approach to body image disturbance

It may be seen from the above that cognitive-behavioural interventions in fields which might be seen as relevant to psychosocial difficulty following disfigurement are potentially powerful, provided that anxiety proves to be a key component of the difficulties faced by disfigured people. In the rest of this chapter, a cognitive-behavioural, fear–avoidance model of psychosocial difficulties following disfigurement is described, including a formulation of factors maintaining the difficulties experienced by sufferers, a rationale for treatment and a number of predictions which may be made from the approach. The model was principally developed in the context of psychological difficulties following facial disfigurement, and this area of client distress will be used as the main example throughout. This form of visible difference is perhaps the most obvious to others, and is therefore a pertinent example through which to explore difficulties with social interactions in particular. The relevance of visibility, as in facial disfigurement, is further illustrated by the interaction of an individual's body image with the social norms of other surrounding bodily appearance. Moreover, it has been argued (Newell 1991, 1999) that the model is more generally applicable both to other forms of disfigurement and to non-disturbed body image. The following chapters will examine the empirical evidence which might be thought to support this model.

The models of body image outlined in Chapter 2 contain within them descriptions of what might be expected in cases of disturbance of that body image. Of the two main models described, it was suggested that Price's (1990a) broad approach, whilst useful and important in nursing, contained a number of flaws, principally circularity of argument and inadequate definition, whilst Slade's (1994) was, by contrast, too narrow, being derived from and applicable principally to eating disorders, whilst concentrating chiefly on perceptual elements of body image and the contribution of the other components to this aspect. However, it was also suggested that the Slade approach could be expanded to include both normal body image and difficulties other than eating disorders. This broadening of the Slade model included reference to Lethem *et al.*'s (1983) fear–avoidance model of exaggerated pain perception, a model with many elements in common with that of Slade, who was, in fact, part of the Lethem *et al.* group (Slade *et al.* 1983).

The Lethem *et al.* (1983) model provides a useful starting point for the cognitive-behavioural approach to facial disfigurement to be described in this chapter. Lethem *et al.* (1983) proposed that people who make adequate recovery from illness (in particular chronic pain) are those who tend to exhibit confrontation rather than avoidance, and that the tendency to confront rather than avoid is determined by interacting factors from the individual's background and environment (see Figure 3.1). The key contributing elements (fear of pain, life events, personality, pain history and coping strategies) produce a *psychosocial context* for the pain event which determines the individual's response to it along a continuum from avoidance to confrontation, and, by extension, from recovery to handicap. Since they were working principally with back pain patients when they devised the model, confrontation and avoidance are described mainly in terms of pain-related activity, and the consequences of avoidance are examined chiefly in terms of changes to the body and failure to rehabilitate physically. However, the key element in the model is that avoidance takes place *because of fear of pain, rather than because of pain itself*. The patient *predicts* that pain is likely to occur if a particular behaviour is performed, and consequently avoids that behaviour. Similarly, if an activity is being performed and the patient predicts that pain is likely to ensue, then that activity will be ceased. Cognitive-behavioural accounts of the genesis and maintenance of anxiety through passive and active avoidance predict that, in consequence, the range of permissible activities will become more and more restricted, and increasingly innocuous stimuli will be interpreted as threatening. Strict behaviourists will attribute these occurrences chiefly to the processes of generalisation and discrimination, and of negative reinforcement of avoidance (Walker 1984). Whilst a number of cognitive interpretations are possible, perhaps the most relevant is derived from Bandura's self-efficacy theory (1977b), which states that the likelihood of an individual performing an activity is based not only on reinforcement but also on the individual's perception of their ability to carry out the activity. Repeated avoidance not only decreases the opportunity for reinforcement, but lowers the individual's perception that the activity is within their capability. In the context of back pain, Lethem *et al.* (1983) note the importance of physical changes resulting from avoidance, such as increased weight and decreased muscle tone. Moreover, a number of psychological changes, such as failure to calibrate pain and increased responsiveness to reinforcement of invalid status, are likely to arise, as the range of perceived abilities decreases. The model is related to the three systems model of Lang (1971), above, and in particular to the notion of desynchrony between the three systems (Rachman and Hodgson 1974). In essence, this model argues that client difficulties are due to such desynchrony. For example, a phobic person in a feared situation might misinterpret relatively mild autonomic symptoms of arousal as indicators of some catastrophic occurrence, such as heart attack, indicating desynchrony between the autonomic and cognitive system. In the case of the Lethem *et al.* (1983) approach, the desynchrony is between the physiological aspects of pain, on the one hand, and the subjective and behavioural aspects on the other. In Lethem *et al.*'s (1983) model, the key element said to maintain and increase disability and pain perception is not the pain itself, but the *fear* of that pain.

A test of the model (Rose *et al.* 1992) demonstrated significant differences between recovered and non-recovered patients. Moreover, some of these differences held good across three different pain problems (post-herpetic neuralgia, low back pain and reflex sympathetic dystrophy), suggesting that the applicability of the model is not restricted to types of pain associated with physical activity.

As we shall see in Chapters 5, 6 and 7, avoidance and anxiety may be widespread amongst sufferers from facial disfigurement. For example, Gamba *et al.* (1992) report avoidance of examining operation sites and looking in mirrors by head and neck cancer patients, whilst complaints of social difficulty are the most frequently reported difficulties amongst disfigured people (Macgregor 1951; Malt 1980; Kalick *et al.* 1981; Rumsey 1983; Rubinow *et al.* 1987; Partridge *et al.* 1994; Robinson *et al.* 1996). Furthermore, good social skills have been found to be the best predictor of adjustment in one study (Kapp-Simon *et al.* 1992). Social skills training has shown promise in increasing well-being and social competence amongst facially disfigured people (Feigenbaum 1981; Robinson *et al.* 1996).

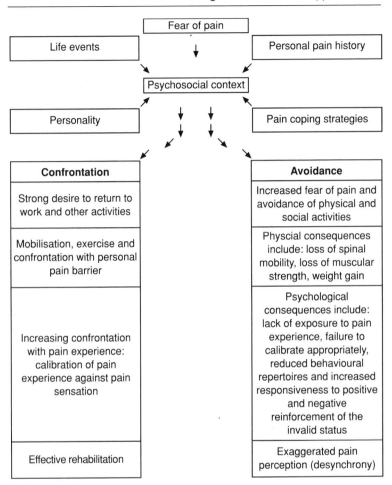

Figure 3.1 Lethem *et al.*'s model of exaggerated pain perception (after Lethem *et al.* 1983)

Newell (1991) has offered a cognitive-behavioural approach to body image disturbance which draws on clinical studies of phobic disorders in general and body dysmorphic disorder (BDD) in particular, and upon conditioning accounts of phobias, the fear–avoidance model of exaggerated pain perception (Lethem *et al.* 1983), the three systems model of Lang (1971) and the social learning and self-efficacy theories of Bandura (1977a, 1977b). Since these constructs are themselves largely convergent, it is perhaps best to see Newell's (1991) formulation of body image difficulties as being derived from Lethem *et al.* (1983). As discussed earlier, this is itself similar to Slade's (1994) model of body image. Newell (1991) assumes many of the psychological difficulties of people who have suffered a threat to body image are similar to those suffered by phobics. In other words, these difficulties are mediated primarily by fear and avoidance, which are themselves primarily maintained by conditioning and the dysfunctional thoughts which often accompany avoidance learning in phobias (Butler 1989). Newell's (1991) cognitive-behavioural formulation asserts that, for disfigured people, activities associated with the lost or damaged part of the body are avoided, because they have been found to give rise to autonomic features of anxiety and to anxiety-provoking thoughts. Furthermore, activities which remind the person of the lost or damaged area, even though not directly associated with it, are likewise avoided. For example, a person might, following mastectomy, avoid reading women's magazines in which articles about cancer, breast augmentation, swimsuits or lingerie might be present. Similarly thoughts associated with the damaged area are resisted, since they also come to be associated with autonomic arousal and anxiety. The process proposed in the 1991 paper for the development of disturbed body image is presented in Figure 3.2.

This formulation required refinement, expansion and testing, because of limitations in its original construction and lack of empirical tests. The 1991 article makes no reference to *how* its formulation might be related to Lethem *et al.*'s (1983) model, and only mentions the development of disturbance. It will be remembered that Lethem *et al.* describe a psychosocial context comprising a number of elements which lead to either disturbance or recovery. It was suggested in Newell (1999) that this psychosocial context is equally applicable to body image, with the following amendments. In this refinement of the 1991 model, 'pain history' was replaced with 'history of changes to body image', following Slade's (1994) model of body image in eating disorders. In a similar way, 'fear of pain' was changed to 'fear of changed body and reactions of others'. This amendment reflects the likelihood that disfigured people may share the same cultural and social norms related to body image as the rest of society, which in turn might contribute to a negative appraisal by disfigured people of their own changed body part. Additionally, the concern of disfigured people with the responses of others is reflected in this amended element. 'Pain coping strategies' was changed, in Newell (1999), to 'body image coping strategies', reflecting the ways in which people have learnt to deal with changes to or imperfections in the body in the past. Lethem *et al.* (1983) also propose two ends of a continuum

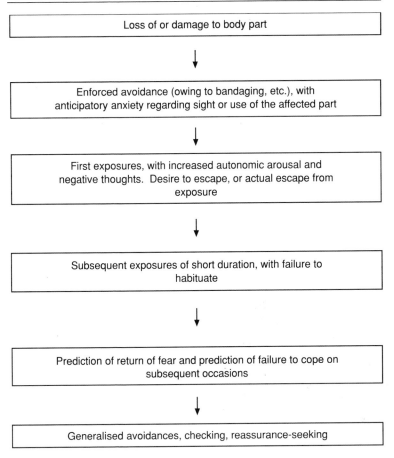

Figure 3.2 A model of disturbed body image (from Newell 1991)

of *results* of pain events: confrontation (and recovery) or avoidance (and chronicity). The process shown in Figure 3.2 should be regarded as an adaptation of the description of the consequences of avoidance in chronic pain described in the Lethem *et al.* article. By contrast, confrontation (or exposure) is associated with a body image which is not disturbed (i.e. which does not interfere with physical and psychological functioning (Goin and Goin 1981)). This process of successful adaptation through confrontation is outlined in Figure 3.3. The fear–avoidance model of response to disfigurement was originated to account for difficulties following insults to body image as a result of surgery, trauma or disease,

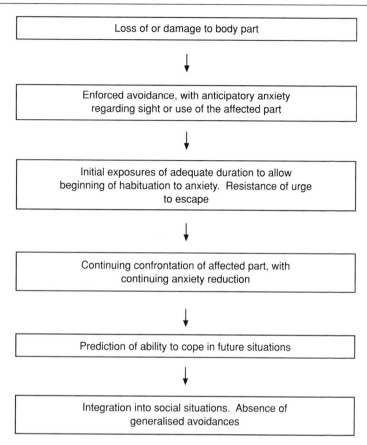

Figure 3.3 A model of successful adaptation following change of body image

and Figure 3.3 therefore represents an account of successful adaptation following such insults. In a slightly altered form, the model accounts equally well for such occurrences and for body image disturbance resulting from disfigurement from birth. In this latter case, since the disfigurement is present from birth, the potential for confrontation or avoidance likewise exists from this time, rather than from the time of occurrence of disfigurement at some later date. Therefore, in the case of the person disfigured from birth, elements of the psychosocial context of disfigurement do not pre-date the occurrence of disfigurement. Indeed, the disfigurement itself may be a major contributing factor in the psychosocial development of the individual. Moreover, elements such as enforced avoidance, which may be present following injury, will be unlikely to be a major factor. Figure 3.4 reflects the most recent version of the fear–avoidance model (Newell 1999).

Figure 3.4 illustrates the particular role of social avoidance. However, this is not intended to be regarded as the sole aspect of avoidance, but was in Newell (1999) offered purely as an illustration. This illustration is, nevertheless, particularly relevant because of the potentially damaging consequences of social avoidance across a broad range of activities. Newell (1999) also suggested that other avoidances (for example of grooming, looking in mirrors, exposing or using the affected part) are associated with anxiety in the same way and have similar kinds of consequences in terms of limitation of the individual's life and disturbance of body image. If we look, for example, at the behaviour of BDD sufferers,

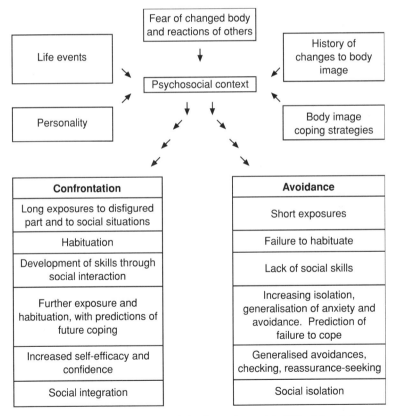

Figure 3.4 A fear–avoidance model of psychosocial difficulties following disfigurement (from Newell 1999)

we see a great deal of anxiety and specific avoidances, albeit in the context of the overvalued idea, and these avoidances are a source of significant handicap to the sufferer. Just as the notion of *fear* of pain and consequent avoidance are the key aspects of Lethem *et al.*'s (1983) fear–avoidance model of exaggerated pain perception, the Newell (1999) fear–avoidance model of psychosocial difficulty following disfigurement has as its central feature *fear* of the changed body and the responses of others. The *actual* responses of people to the disfigured individual are doubtless often negative, but this does not alter the model presented here. Just as Lethem *et al.* (1983) recognise the role of others in maintaining avoidance behaviour in the person with chronic pain, so the Newell (1999) model accepts the role of others in maintaining the psychosocial difficulties of disfigured people. Indeed, the reactions of such people are likely to have a profound effect in terms of increasing the disfigured person's fear of such reactions. Nevertheless, it is suggested that such fear is likely to lessen with continuing exposure and to increase with avoidance. One purpose of the fear–avoidance model is to offer an account which differentiates between those who adjust well in the face of the inappropriate actions of others and those who do not.

The expanded account of fear and avoidance as possible mediators in disturbed body image is potentially useful. For example, it is possible that this model may be capable of accounting for the psychosocial difficulties experienced by a broad range of disfigured people, regardless of the specific cause of their disfigurement. As we noted earlier, the theoretical and practical grounding of the model in the cognitive-behavioural approach to phobias and anxiety is a potential strength, since this approach has received considerable support from both clinical and laboratory studies of the acquisition of fears and phobias (Marks 1987). In this context, it is instructive that the avoidances described by social phobics are similar to anecdotal accounts of many of the social difficulties of sufferers from disfigurement. If the formulation proves robust, there are immediate consequences in terms of interventions with disfigured people. These may be as diverse as preparation for surgery, recovery from disfiguring trauma and surgery, work with children disfigured since birth at the level of cognitive and social development, and interventions with people actively suffering the psychological consequences of disfigurement.

Whilst this is encouraging, it should be emphasised that the approach possesses the great weakness that it has been, until recently, like Price's (1990a, 1990b) model, almost entirely speculative. There have, for example, been no treatment reports of an approach based on the fear–

avoidance model with disfigured people. Papers which have suggested that exposure might be important in addressing disfigurement (e.g. Tarrier and Maguire 1984; Price 1986, 1990a; Griffiths 1990) are few and are rarely accompanied by evidence. The Rumsey/Partridge group, who do provide encouraging initial evidence of effectiveness, do not clearly report the contribution of specific instructions in exposure to their skills training-oriented package.

Not only is the use of cognitive-behavioural interventions based on exposure principles for people with facial disfigurements itself speculative, but the assumption that the clinical picture of disfigured individuals will be similar to those for whom cognitive-behavioural interventions have been effective (e.g. social phobics, agoraphobics, BDD sufferers) is itself a matter for empirical investigation. For example, Latham (1997) has noted that BDD sufferers are by definition different from disfigured individuals, since they lack any visible deformity. The similarity or otherwise of these groups may usefully be investigated before further acceptance of the fear–avoidance approach. The presence or otherwise of avoidance perhaps represents a practically important difficulty for the model. We have, until recently, had no evidence that the undoubted avoidances described in first-hand accounts, anecdotal reports and small studies are actually socially phobic or agoraphobic in nature. In other words, we did not know whether or not these avoidances were maintained through a *fear* of entering social or public situations, which is in turn related to expectations about ability to cope in such situations. In the case of social phobics and disfigured people, such work has now been undertaken (Newell 2000; Newell and Marks 2000) and is reported in Chapter 7. By the same token, it should be noted that there is no reason to suppose that disfigured people have an overvalued idea related to their appearance. Although individual attitude may well play a part in reaction to disfigurement, as it clearly does in BDD, this is unlikely to reach the level of importance it does in BDD. However, this lack of concordance is necessarily a problem for the fear–avoidance model. Even though the model was derived in part from clinical work with this group, the key point of similarity between BDD sufferers and disfigured people is seen as the anxiety and avoidance which it is suggested they share. Equally, it may be noted from the literature that disfigured people report being preoccupied with the responses of others to their appearance. Arguments about whether it is important that this preoccupation does or does not constitute an overvalued idea, given that disfigured people do indeed have visible deformity, may be more of theoretical than of therapeutic importance. The central issue is, arguably, whether disfigured people, like social phobics and BDD sufferers, experience avoidance and negative thoughts which are ameliorated by similar interventions. Work on investigating this proposition has now begun (Newell 1998; Newell and Clarke 2000) and suggests that exposure is indeed a promising intervention (see Chapter 7). Taken together, the findings that facially disfigured people resemble social phobics, experience anxiety in social situations and avoid such situations, and respond to cognitive-behavioural intervention represent considerable preliminary support for the model.

The model described above was developed with a clear clinical aim in view: the amelioration of the psychosocial difficulties experienced by disfigured people. As a consequence, it is, like the models of Lethem *et al.* (1983) and Slade (1994), primarily a model of the development of *disturbance*. Within all these models, including Newell (1998, 1999), the development of *non-problematic* behaviours and experiences is also examined. The account of how these non-problematic behaviours and experiences are derived from the various elements of the model, and the way these elements combine to attempt to predict responses to threat, offers us a way of accounting for how body image develops in the *absence of serious threat* also. For example, we may conclude, from Figure 3.4, that a non-disturbed body image will arise from a psychosocial context which leads the person to pursue tactics which involve, as habits of thought and behaviour, the confrontation of changes to body image, and attempts to adapt to such changes. Such changes need not involve the considerable levels of difficulty we might expect to be associated with disfigurement. On the contrary, many will be seen as part of normal development (for example, growth, minor illness and injury in childhood, development of body hair, and so on). The development of a non-problematic (i.e. that which does not interfere with physical and psychological functioning (Goin and Goin 1981)) body image will involve successfully meeting these developmental challenges, through the use of these confrontational tactics, which will in turn feed once again into the psychosocial context, as part of the person's body image history and coping tactics.

Exercise

Investigate the three systems theory of human experience yourself. Perhaps there is some activity which causes you anxiety. For example, many people fear public speaking. It may even be that you have a mild phobia (say of spiders or insects). Identify the fear which is most relevant to yourself, but remember this should *not* be so great as to cause you *considerable* anxiety. The aim of this exercise is to find out something about the nature of the CB approach, *not* to embark on a programme of tackling a clinical phobia through cognitive-behaviour therapy. If you have such a phobia (and many do), and it causes you distress in daily life (and for many it does *not*) *and* you want to tackle it, there are many self-help books available. One is suggested in the reading list for Chapter 8. However, that is a project for another day. For this exercise, concentrate on mild to moderate fear.

Now, make a date in your diary when you will confront the fear. For example, agree with your ward manager that you will give a formal presentation to all the ward staff on some aspect of your work. Keep a note *before, during and after* the event of what you experience physically, what thoughts you think and what you do. These last three elements are the three systems.

You may well experience physical symptoms of anxiety, negative thoughts about your abilities, a desire to leave the situation, or you may avoid talking in much detail. At the end of the event, you will probably feel a *rapid* reduction in the physical feelings and other negative experiences. This is like what happens when phobic people enter and escape from feared situations, although for them the level of discomfort is often much greater, and, in consequence, the amount of relief on escape is also greater.

You may well also note, if the event lasts for long enough (say over 20–30 minutes), that you experience a *gradual* reduction in the negative experiences, even though you remain in the situation. This is the process of habituation described earlier in this chapter, and the process by which much cognitive-behaviour therapy works.

Key further reading

Fonagy, A. and Roth, P. (1996) *What Works for Whom*. New York: Guilford.
  A fairly comprehensive review of the effectiveness of various psychotherapies. Particularly interesting given that, whilst the authors are by no means wedded to the cognitive-behavioural approach, this approach still makes an extremely strong showing.

Hawton, K., Salkovskis, P.M., Kirk, J. and Clark, D.M. (eds) (1989) *Cognitive-Behaviour Therapy for Psychiatric Problems. A Practical Guide*. Oxford: Oxford University Press.
  Comprehensive general guide to the techniques of the cognitive-behavioural approach to a range of client difficulties. Good chapter on social phobia.

Marks, I.M. (1987) *Fears, Phobias and Rituals.* New York: Oxford University Press.

Excellent, but very detailed, text book examining clinical features and treatment of anxiety disorders from a cognitive-behavioural perspective.

Part 2

Disfigurement and its consequences

Chapter 4

Disfigurement and stigma

This chapter begins by exploring general aspects of disfigurement, disability and stigma, as well as examining the potential size of the problem of disfigurement and its psychosocial consequences. It then offers some developmental context to the problems of disfigurement through a brief examination of children's experiences of disfigurement, whilst a final section considers early qualitative studies of disfigured people's experiences, and accounts by disfigured people themselves. Although unsystematised, these accounts provide ample testimony to the difficulties faced by disfigured individuals in response both to threats to their body image and to the inappropriate behaviour of others.

Frances Macgregor (1951) noted that less attention is paid by researchers to disfigurement than to other forms of handicap. Nevertheless, she believed, the problems faced by this group might at least be the equal of those experiencing other bodily impairments. As with many of the examples used in this book, Macgregor's area of work concerned facial disfigurement. She noted that the face has profound social significance, and that the attitudes and prejudices of society towards those of atypical appearance are both negative and potentially of great consequence to the sufferer. The majority of her respondents' complaints related to their social interactions with others.

Disfigurement as disability

Whilst the disabling effects of disfigurement may not be immediately obvious, it seems clear from the literature that researchers either explicitly or implicitly examine disfigurement in the context of disability, drawing, for example, on the concept of stigma of disabled people to account for attitudes to disfigured individuals and examining social, psychological and behavioural consequences in terms of impairment of functioning.

Disfigured people themselves often report the consequences of their disfigurement in terms of such impaired functioning. The Office of Population Censuses and Surveys' examination of disability in the UK (Martin *et al.* 1988), outlining patterns of disability based on a national survey, defined disfigurement as disability if an individual 'suffers from a scar, blemish or deformity which severely affects ability to lead a normal life'. They report a total prevalence of 9 per 1000 in the population, which breaks down by age as follows: age 16 to 59 – 5 per 1000; age 60 to 74 – 18 per 1000; age 75 and above – 27 per 1000. They estimate the total number of sufferers within the population as 391,000 (age 16 to 59 – 163,000; age 60 to 74 – 141,000; age 75 and over – 87,000). A global assessment of impairment of performance was presented, and is shown in Table 4.1.

A limitation of the survey is that site of the disfigurement is not recorded. Thus, we may not examine whether disfigurement of one area led to more impairment than another. However, the number of people affected is clearly substantial, with the obvious consequences for the nation, in terms of both economic burden and human suffering. The tendency to consider different bodily areas of disfigurement together is an abiding problem within the literature, and gives rise to difficulties both in conducting a review of the area and in arriving at reliable estimates of the extent of the problem. For example, in this book, a good deal of material related to burns injuries is covered, since such injuries represent a considerable source of disfigurement. However, many of the studies

Table 4.1 Impairment of performance by disfigurement according to age: frequency at each level (% of disabled people with disfigurement as their disability)

	Severity level					Total (all severity
	1–2*	*3–4*	*5–6*	*7–8*	*9–10*	levels)†
All ages	4	6	7	11	16	7
16–59	7	8	9	13	19	9
60–74	4	7	8	12	20	7
75 and over	2	2	4	8	12	4

Source: Martin *et al.* (1988).

Notes

*Severity is defined as the extent to which an individual's performance is limited by impairment. 10 = most severe.

†Total percentages are not simple summations of category percentages because the base samples vary across severity levels.

do not differentiate between the areas burned, with the result that any conclusions drawn from such studies about reaction to disfigurement in terms of psychosocial adjustment are at best tentative, since impairment of function may be as important a feature as the disfigurement. The same issue applies in other areas. For example, people who have undergone surgery for oral cancer may experience difficulties in social settings as much from the practical difficulties involved in, say, talking and eating, as from changes in appearance. This is problematic for the consideration of the impact of disfigurement, but also if we are attempting to differentiate between the respective roles played in body image and its disturbance by function and appearance.

Disability, disfigurement and stigma

Numerous commentators have suggested that disfigured people are stigmatised persons. In an early review of the effects of stigma and of other psychosocial sequelae of disability, Barker (1948) suggests that the effects of an unusual appearance have preoccupied people for many years. He notes that Francis Bacon had stated that 'deformed people are commonly vengeful – returning in coin the evil that nature has visited upon them'. Although this is clearly an anecdotal opinion from well before the beginning of systematised examination of disfigurement, or indeed of disability and illness in general, it is, however, an interesting early example of negative stereotyping of disfigured people. The use of the word 'evil' in this context is likewise instructive, suggesting the commonly held belief that physical beauty is good, and deformity bad. Interestingly, this age-old belief still persists today, and some empirical investigation of it has been undertaken by psychologists (Landy and Sigall 1974; Benson et al. 1976).

Barker (1948) also suggests that disabled people occupy a similar situation in society to other despised groups such as Negroes and Jews. His assertion was not demonstrated at that time, but has been cited by subsequent authors in support of the inclusion of disfigured people under the category of stigmatised minority groups (e.g. Goffman 1963), and later studies have indeed confirmed the existence of both prejudice against and stigmatisation of disfigured people.

Stigma were originally marks deliberately inflicted on slaves (Goffman 1963) so that others would be aware of their station in life. Goffman's (1963) collection of essays about stigma and stigmatised people has influenced researchers in the field of disfigurement (e.g. Rumsey 1983). He combines a number of groups (e.g. criminals, disfigured people, ethnic and religious groups) under the heading of stigmatised people and defines stigma as the situation whereby an individual is 'disqualified from full social acceptance'. Goffman (1963) distinguishes between two categories of person: *the discredited* – those whose stigmatised status is readily apparent to others (who respond to it), and *the discreditable* – those whose status is not apparent, but towards whom others would respond with stigmatisation if it were. For most purposes, disfigured individuals fall into the former category, since perceptibility is regarded as a crucial aspect of stigmatisation. This should, however, be distinguished from obtrusiveness – the degree to which the stigma obtrudes upon our interactions with stigmatised persons. Thus, disfigured people are discredited because their disfigurement is both visible and, since it is liable to interfere with social intercourse (for example, by interfering with eye contact because people stare at it or seek to avoid looking at the face), obtrusive. Goffman (1963) also asserts that stigmatised people share with 'normals' their views of the significance of the stigma, since they have incorporated the standards of society as a whole.

Goffman (1963) describes the role of control of information by the stigmatised person in maintenance of personal identity. This control relates to such issues as being able to pass as non-stigmatised in certain situations. Considerable effort seems to go into such control of information, and members of stigmatised groups are often concerned about being discovered.

The ability to control information about stigmatised group membership is obviously limited for disfigured people, but does yield an interesting speculation about behavioural avoidance. In a discussion about the nature of perceptibility, Goffman (1963) notes that the stigmatisation of race becomes invisible under certain circumstances, for example during telephone conversations and in writing. Interactions of this kind represent one way in which disfigured people might seek to control information about their disfigured status, through avoidance of face-to-face contact. The use of camouflage tactics such as make-up and particular clothing may represent a similar attempt. By contrast, Goffman (1963) notes that disclosure of stigmatised status, for example through deliberate wearing of stigma symbols, may enable the use of adaptive actions by the stigmatised person. The potential power of wearing of such symbols is increased when people who are supportive of the stigmatised group respond by sharing the symbol.

Goffman also notes the use by stigmatised individuals of in-group and out-group alignments. The in-group is the group to which an individual naturally belongs. In-group alignment is reported as more characteristic of politicised movements, such as those of different ethnic groups, who seek to gain self-esteem through this identification. The spread of in-group alliance to groups such as psychiatric patients and ex-patients, disabled people and disfigured people is comparatively recent, and may become important to the cessation of avoidance behaviours amongst disfigured people.

Whilst disclosure tactics may help adaptation, the status and adjustment of the stigmatised person, particularly in the absence of a strong in-group to which to relate, are also likely to be mediated by the responses of the out-group. Novak and Lerner (1968) hypothesised that people stare at handicapped individuals because they fear the disability could happen to them. This in turn violates their belief in a 'just world' where individuals are responsible for and in control of their fates. Violation of this belief leads to dysphoria, since it is uncomfortable to live in a world where events are random. In order to maintain their belief in a just world, people then derogate/stigmatise the disabled person.

In a study of helping behaviour and stigma, Piliavin et al. (1975) investigated the role of their two stage model of helping behaviour in predicting responses to facially disfigured people in an emergency situation. They were able to demonstrate that it was the physical stimulus of the stigma (a port wine stain) which led to a decrease in helping behaviour, rather than any perceived feared consequence of intervention or attribution of reprehensibility to the victim in the simulated emergency which constituted their investigation. It might be that refraining from helping represents, via avoidance of an anxiety-provoking interaction, a way of decreasing the arousal created by violation of the 'just world' belief.

The above accounts of stigmatisation of disabled and disfigured people might be said to share a single broad feature: the desire to maintain comfort or to decrease uncomfortable arousal in the presence of the untoward stimulus of disfigurement. An alternative to the notion of stigma/derogation as an explanation of bias against disabled or facially disfigured individuals is advanced by Langer et al. (1976). They propose that people stare at disfigured or disabled people not because they derogate them, but because disabled people represent novel stimuli, which elicit exploratory behaviour in order to render the world more regular and, thus, predictable and safer. The discomfort experienced by people in the presence of physically atypical individuals derives, according to Langer et al. (1976), from a contradiction between the desire to stare and the general social prohibition against staring. In a now classic study, they reported three experiments: two involved the examination of photographs in a picture gallery, whilst the third involved interacting with either a disabled or non-disabled person.

In their first experiment, fifteen male and fifteen female subjects viewed photographs of a normal, a pregnant and an obviously disabled woman in a photographic gallery. Since photographs are intended to be looked at, no social norm is thus offended. Female subjects were significantly more likely to look at the disabled woman than the pregnant woman, and least likely to look at the normal. In male subjects, the normal woman and the disabled woman were equally likely to be looked at. The authors speculate that the novelty of the disabled woman was equalled, for men, by their desire to look at an 'attractive normal female' (Langer *et al.* 1976).

The second experiment, using male subjects only, expanded on the first by manipulating the sanction on staring, through the introduction of an observer. Forty males looked at photographs of a normal male and a hunchback whilst an observer (apparently another viewer in the gallery) was present on 50% of occasions. Subjects spent significantly more time observing the hunchbacked man when alone, but significantly more time observing the normal man when observed, thus offering support for the notion that desire to stare at a novel stimulus is suppressed by the perception of a social norm against staring as represented by the presence of another person.

In the final experiment, thirty-six male and thirty-six female subjects interacted with a pregnant, normal or apparently disabled confederate, with or without prior exposure to the stimulus person via a one-way screen. Subjects sat significantly further away from the most novel stimulus (the disabled person) and from those stimulus persons to whom they had not had access. The two variables interacted, so that distances were virtually the same for all levels of the novel stimulus condition when prior exposure had been given. The authors state that they found no evidence of derogation, as assessed by a measure of liking. However, this is rather weak evidence for the absence of derogation, since responses to a pen and paper test could merely have been ones perceived by subjects as socially acceptable.

The first two experiments offer quite convincing evidence for the novel stimulus hypothesis, but the third is less convincing. Whilst it is indeed encouraging to see that even brief prior exposure to the disabled stimulus person led to greater physical proximity, Langer *et al.*'s (1976) novel stimulus hypothesis is not necessary to account for this. If we assume that greater proximity represented decreased discomfort in the presence of the stimulus person, this *might* result from decreased contradiction between the desire to stare at a (no longer novel) stimulus and desire not to contravene the social norm against staring. However, this greater proximity is equally explicable in conditioning terms. Individuals with prior exposure have had an opportunity to habituate to the uncomfortable arousal caused by violation of the 'just world' beliefs posited by Novak and Lerner (1968). Of course, habituation is itself a phenomenon consequent upon decreasing novelty of a stimulus, but is a much more basic, physiological process than that implied by the novel stimulus hypothesis, since the component of conflict between desire to stare and desire for conformity with the social norm against staring is not required by the conditioning account.

The authors suggest that discomfort and avoidance applied to physically stigmatised people has in the past been confused with derogation. Whilst it is quite possibly the case that, as the authors suggest, novelty needs to be taken into account to fully understand stigmatisation, it is not accurate to state that derogation of physically stigmatised people does not occur. As we shall see later in this chapter, accounts of negative verbal and non-verbal behaviours in response to facially disfigured people are frequent.

It is worth noting, in conclusion to the examination of the role of stigma in disfigurement, that the elements of Novak and Lerner's (1968) fear/arousal and Langer et al.'s (1976) novel stimulus accounts might both be usefully and economically explained by Gray's (1982a, 1982b) description of the role of the hippocampus and septal area in regulating autonomic arousal. This account hypothesises the existence of a 'comparator' within the hippocampus, whose role is to compare 'stored regularities' about the environment within the brain with occurrences in the actual environment, and to detect the occurrence of mismatches between the two. In the event of such mismatches, behaviour is inhibited, arousal and attention are increased, and control over a number of behaviours passes to the autonomic nervous system, in preparation for fight or flight, giving rise to what is often construed, in psychological disorder, as anxiety. If we accept that disfigured people represent novel stimuli, we might speculate that Gray's (1982a, 1982b) comparator detects a mismatch between the stored regularities of what constitutes normal human physiognomy and the actual example of a disfigured person. This, in turn, leads to anxiety and to a series of related behaviours such as avoidances and derogation.

In this context, it is interesting to note that habituation leads to a decrease in such anxieties as phobias and compulsions (Marks 1987), which are believed by Gray (1982a, 1982b) to be mediated by the comparator. Since the key components of phobias and compulsions are avoidance and repetitive behaviours such as checking respectively, it is tempting to speculate once again that habituation is the mechanism responsible for the decreased avoidance behaviour shown to disabled people following exposure in Langer *et al.*'s third experiment. Habituation might also lead to a decrease of derogation (if this is viewed as a kind of cognitive avoidance (Williams *et al.* 1988)) or, indeed, of staring behaviour, if this is viewed as a form of checking ritual.

Whilst these comments are highly speculative, Kleck *et al.* (1966) did find increased autonomic arousal in the presence of a handicapped rather than a non-handicapped confederate, regardless of whether subjects described themselves as uncomfortable in the presence of the handicapped individual, again suggesting a relatively simple physiological underpinning to some responses to disfigured people, although it is unlikely that a conditioning account will ever offer a full explanation of these complex interactions.

Disfigurement and stigma in children

Early studies indicate that unattractive children are apparently disadvantaged from an early age (Dion 1973; Landy and Sigall 1974; Rich 1975). With increasing age, children show bias towards competence and aversion to physical disability (Sigelman and Singleton 1986), whilst Richman and Eliason (1982) suggest parents and teachers have lower expectations of facially disfigured children. A study specifically of children with craniofacial abnormalities (Field and Vega-Lahr 1984) offered evidence that mothers of such children are less active during interactions with their infants than mothers of normal children at age 3 months.

Barden *et al.* (1989) argue that corrective surgical intervention with disfigured children will improve interactions. The argument assumes: that the infant–caregiver relationship is a key determinant of psychological adjustment and personality development into adulthood; that physical attractiveness is a demonstrated determinant of later success in social relationships; that craniofacially abnormal children are rated at the bottom of the attractiveness continuum prior to surgery. Barden *et al.* (1989) examined mother–child interactions and self-report ratings of maternal general life and parental satisfaction, involving five mother-infant dyads where the children had a craniofacial abnormality and five where they did not. Mothers of children with craniofacial abnormalities were consistently less nurturant – mothers of non-disfigured children scored more positively overall on every measure and on 26 of 27 possible individual comparisons. The authors also found significantly less tactile/ kinetic stimulation, less affectionate touching, less time demonstrating a toy, less holding of the child in a face-to-face position, and less responsivity to behavioural cues. The children with craniofacial abnormalities themselves touched their parents less and were less likely to smile/laugh and less responsive to mothers. However, the mothers of craniofacially abnormal children reported being more satisfied with parenting than the mothers of non-disfigured children, and reported more positive life events after pregnancy.

The authors wonder whether the discrepancy they found between self-report and observation is a time-limited coping mechanism or is indicative of subsequent dysfunction. They note that not holding in face-to-face contact limits chances of reinforcement of the mother by infant smiling and that craniofacially abnormal children smile less and so may be less able to give reinforcement. They suggest that such children may be less socially responsive to caregivers, and so mothers' attempts at nurturing go unrewarded and thus decrease in frequency.

Whilst this is a small study, from which any conclusions must be extremely limited, it is nevertheless potentially important because the observational element was well conducted, and, despite the extremely small groups, considerable differences were noticeable simply from visual inspection of the data. However, it should be noted first that the discrepancy between observations and self-reports is not necessarily important, since it may have been caused by a social desirability response, and the observational element has low ecological validity owing to its short duration and artificial situation. The raters were not blind to the condition of the experiment, and may well have applied biased ratings to the interactions of the dyads including craniofacially abnormal children. Finally, the authors' suggestions regarding the non-reinforcing behaviours of the children are highly speculative, not only because of the size of the groups, but also because the alternative argument (that mothers do not reinforce craniofacially abnormal children, whose own interactive behaviour is thus extinguished) is equally persuasive, but is not mentioned.

Children express a preference for attractive peers at an early age (Dion 1973) and also notice disfigurement from early in childhood (Conant and Budoff 1983). The preference of children for attractive peers is apparently reflected in their attitudes towards facially disfigured people. Rumsey *et al.* (1986a) examined children between the ages of 5 and 11 in an attempt to observe the age at which stereotyping of facially disfigured individuals commenced. Using before/after photographs of adults who had received facial surgery for minor facial abnormalities, they asked children to choose either 'before' or 'after' photographs in response to positive and negative questions regarding the potential stimulus persons. Whilst younger children chose at a chance level, 11-year-olds chose in the stereotyped direction at a rate of 75%, choosing 'before' photographs in response to negative questions and 'after' photographs in response to positive questions. Moreover, female photographs received more stereotyping than male, suggesting that facial disfigurement in females is a greater cause of negative reactions than in males.

The authors of this carefully conducted study conclude that there may not be stereotyping against facially deformed people until after age 11. However, it may be wise to be cautious in accepting this finding. Children discriminate with regard to attractiveness from a young age (Dion 1973) and, although studies of attractiveness generally do not include disfigured stimulus persons, such individuals are often reported as being less attractive (Barden *et al.* 1989). Furthermore, the authors note that their stimulus photographs showed people whose deformity was a 'minor irregularity of the jaw'. Indeed, the surgery performed upon the target persons amounted only to a revision of the mandible of up to half an inch, without concurrent superficial plastic surgery (Bull and Rumsey 1988). The children might well have shown stereotyping at an earlier age if the level of deformity in the 'before' photographs had been higher.

Moreover, in an element of her 1983 PhD thesis, Rumsey showed 7-year-old ($n = 84$) children male and female non-disfigured, trauma-scarred and birthmark-disfigured adult stimulus photographs, and asked them to compose stories about the individuals shown in the photographs. She carried out content analysis of the resulting stories. Examination of the themes most frequently arising suggested that the children saw disfigured individuals as more likely to be unhappy/nasty people, more likely to assume negative roles in the stories, and possibly (in the case of female stimuli) more likely to be single (Rumsey 1983). These findings seem to suggest that children form stereotyped views of disfigured individuals at an earlier age than that suggested by the Rumsey *et al.* (1986a) study.

It is possible that severity of disfigurement in children is correlated with degree of psychological difficulty. In a study of children with cleft lips and palates, Broder and Strauss (1987) compared thirteen children with cleft lips, thirteen with cleft lip and palates, fourteen with cleft palates and eighteen controls aged from 6 to 9 years with regard to their scores on the Primary Self Concept Inventory, which consists of three domains: personal self, social self and intellectual self.

Subjects with cleft palate only were judged as being of normal appearance by the interviewer. Those with cleft lips had lower self-report scores on the personal, social and total scales than controls, but not lower intellectual scores. Children with cleft palates had lower scores than controls on the social self scale only. No significant differences were found between those with cleft lips and those with cleft palates in any domain. Children with cleft lip and palates scored lower in all domains than controls, and also lower in most domains than those with cleft lips or cleft palates alone.

The authors suggest that these findings support the notion that greater psychological difficulty is found in those with visible rather than invisible defects. However, the results are by no means unequivocal, since the only differences of this kind are between controls and those with defects, not between those with visible and invisible defects. Likewise, the results do not, contrary to the authors' suggestion, fully support a 'beauty is good' hypothesis (see Chapter 5), since those with visible defects do *not* perceive themselves more negatively than those with invisible defects, only more so than controls. Moreover, those with *invisible* defects also perceive themselves more negatively than controls within the social domain, once again not supporting the 'beauty is good' hypothesis. Finally, the authors suggested that their findings showed the stigmatising consequences of facial disfigurement. In fact, they show no such thing, both because of the equivocal nature of the findings themselves, and because stigmatisation was never directly investigated in the study.

A small survey by Noar (1991) of thirty-two patients with cleft lips and palates (mean age 19.9) and their parents shows findings which contrast with those of Broder and Strauss (1987). If we take teasing as an instance of stigmatising behaviour, Noar found that only some 25% of the patients reported having been teased by peers. He also noted that cleft patients have a generally similar body image to normal subjects, with the exception that whilst those with clefts are concerned about the cleft itself, normal subjects tend to be more preoccupied with growth and with stylised standards of beauty. It is, however, difficult to draw direct comparisons between the study samples without knowing how comparable the level of disfigurement was between the two groups.

The tendency for children to show increasing aversion to physical disability with age (Sigelman and Singleton 1986) is perhaps reflected in the experiences of children with facial deformities. Pertschuk and Whitaker (1982) found more disturbed functioning in older children in their sample of fifty-one patients referred for reconstruction of craniofacial abnormalities. Although almost all the children reported teasing, adolescents were markedly more disturbed than younger children. Whilst the authors note that this may have been a procedural artefact arising from the need to use different measures in the two groups, they also stress that corroborating interviews, observed behaviour and parental reports appear to confirm their findings. Alternatively, they suggest younger children may have been better able to deny their problems, although this is clearly not amenable to investigation without both a reliable operationalisation of the concept of denial and a specific element of the study to test for its presence. Surprisingly, though they acknowledge that opposite-sex relationships increase during adolescence, the authors do not stress this as a possible reason for greater difficulties in older children, nor do they mention the likely broadening of social life in adolescence or the lessening of dependence on parents and family. It seems worthwhile to speculate that increased difficulty with age in this sample is a consequence of having to deal with the developmental tasks of adolescence whilst having the additional burden of a facial disfigurement. The authors also report that, in common with some other studies, little correlation was found between level of disfigurement and disturbance.

There is some indication that social skill in disfigured children might be linked to adjustment. Kapp-Simon *et al.* (1992) explored the relationship between self-perception, social skills and adjustment in a study of forty-five young adolescents (mean age 12.3 years) with craniofacial abnormalities. They gave their sample measures of personality and self-perception and a behaviour problem checklist, and found that whilst social skills, self-perception and behavioural inhibition were within the normal range, the average adjustment score was considerably below the average of a normative population. The best predictors of adjustment were social skills and athletic competence. The social skills scores made the only significant impact, however, with athletic competence adding little to the predictive value. The authors concluded that a significant number of children with craniofacial abnormalities were at risk of poor adjustment, and further suggested that improving their social skills might increase their adjustment levels.

Unfortunately, Kapp-Simon *et al.* do not comment upon one important possible confounding element of their study. It could well be the case that the children are better adjusted for some other (uninvestigated) reason, and that this improves their social skills. This is always a problem with drawing inferences from correlational studies, but is particularly problematic in this instance, since there is evidence of reciprocity in social interactions, particularly with regard to the perception of attractive people as more socially skilled, and the possibility that such people indeed possess greater social skills. Since no ratings of the attractiveness of the subjects in the current study were undertaken, varying levels of such attractiveness is one simple possible source of the correlation between social skill and adjustment. We should expect more attractive individuals to have more access to social reinforcement and therefore be more likely to respond with greater skill as a result of more rewarding practice opportunities. This greater social approval might also account for their greater social adjustment, whether or not they showed greater skill.

Although a review by Lefebvre and Arndt (1988) of 15 years of psychiatric consultation in the care of children with facial disfigurement does not specifically comment on the role of social skills in mediating adjustment, it does identify a number of protective factors, including intelligence, positive mood, sense of humour, strong parental marital relationship, family and community support, and personality characteristics. Whilst a number of these factors can be seen as directly or indirectly related to social interaction, the paper is weakened by the fact that only the first two of these asserted protective factors are substantiated by citations. Despite this shortcoming, the assertions of Lefebvre and Arndt are generally consistent with both the Kapp-Simon *et al.* (1992) findings and the few empirical studies of social skills training in adults with disfigurements (see Chapter 6).

Macgregor *et al.* (1953) suggested that mild deformity might be harder to cope with than severe disfigurement. Reich (1969) has speculated that this is because severely deformed individuals can predict adverse responses with more regularity. They are thus more prepared for negative responses than the more mildly disfigured. Whilst this argument is attractive from a conditioning perspective, since we should expect more prolonged and regular exposure to an anxiety-provoking stimulus such as the negative reactions of others to give rise to habituation and, therefore, to anxiety reduction (Walker 1984, 1987), it is not universally supported by the evidence, since more severe disfigurement is sometimes associated with worse psychological adjustment (see Chapter 6).

In an investigation of the contention that less severity of deformity leads to worse psychological adjustment in childhood, Lansdown *et al.* (1991) rated the intelligence, self-concept and behaviour of twenty-seven facially disfigured children, twelve control children, twenty-six siblings and twelve control siblings. The facially disfigured children were classified for deformity according to parental account of amount stared at in public, which accorded significantly with raters' opinions of their photographs.

No significant differences in intelligence were found between the groups. Whilst there was no significant association between severity of disfigurement and scores on the total self-concept scale, a non-significant trend was found for mildly disfigured children to report a lower self-concept on seven items related to appearance and popularity from the scale. There were no differences between the behaviour scale scores of any groups. Significant differences were found between siblings, with siblings of mildly disfigured children showing most disturbances. These siblings were more disturbed than any patients

Despite this, the authors conclude the results support the contention of greater disturbance in mild disfigurement, and posit that this is because more disfigured individuals have learnt to cope with a 'consistent reality' of being stared at, pitied, shunned and insulted, whilst the mildly disfigured might worry about whether their deformity has been noted. This is an intriguing idea, which supports a behavioural explanation based upon habituation. However, the authors present *no* actual evidence for their speculation in this much-cited study. They found no significant differences according to level of deformity, and thus their hypothesis is not supported.

First-hand accounts by disfigured people

Considerable qualitative research has informed both the work of quantitative researchers in the area and the model of body image presented in this book. Indeed, Macgregor, one of the most influential commentators on the plight of disfigured people, approaches her work from the sociological tradition and from a largely qualitative standpoint. Whilst these qualitative studies lack the predictive power of quantitative research, they nevertheless provide a fascinating, detailed account of the experiences of small groups of disfigured individuals, and have been helpful in indicating areas to which more systematic research should be addressed. Similarly, first-hand accounts by disfigured people demonstrate the range and degree of difficulties they experience more forcefully than can quantitative approaches.

This brief section focuses, largely without comment or analysis, on a small selection from the literature of first-hand accounts, in order to demonstrate in detail some of the personal ramifications of the experiences to be summarised in the quantitative studies described in Chapters 5 and 6. The focus of the selection is on social interactions. Although there are a considerable number of brief accounts of personal experiences of disfigurement available, particularly in the popular press, these generally lack detail or depth and are not reported here. This section focuses particularly on the work of one respected qualitative researcher, Frances Macgregor, who has been active in disfigurement research for over 40 years, and on two well-known, detailed first-hand accounts from the UK. General themes from the selections are then summarised.

In her earliest major contribution to the area, Macgregor (Macgregor 1951; Macgregor et al. 1953) interviewed seventy-four plastic surgery patients suffering from four levels of deformity. Whilst a number of structured psychological tests were used and reported, most of the work involved qualitative reports of the interview content, from which Macgregor identified themes such as social disadvantage, expectancies, modes of response and adjustment. In particular, Macgregor et al. (1953) offered four case histories representing the four levels of disfigurement identified in the study. Whilst the material is presented in a highly integrated way, so that it is often difficult to distinguish between results from various elements of the empirical work and comments on the work of earlier commentators and research projects, considerable use is made of direct quotes from sufferers, many of which attest to the degree of social performance difficulty, isolation and stigma experienced. The following are illustrative examples:

> People think I'm a tough character because I talk out of the side of my mouth.
>
> I avoid restaurants as people may think I have a disease and won't want to eat with me.
>
> (Macgregor et al. 1953: 71)

> Children would make fun of the way I looked and say I wasn't normal.
>
> People seem to think I've changed because my face has.
>
> (Macgregor et al. 1953: 72)

> When I have an appointment with a new contact, I try to manage by standing at a distance and facing the door, so the person entering will have more time to see me and get adjusted to my face before we start talking.
>
> (Macgregor et al. 1953: 85)

Before [plastic surgery], when I was with people I used to put so much energy into putting on an act and pretending I was happy when I wasn't.

(Macgregor *et al.* 1953: 90)

The above examples illustrate the impact of disfigurement on sufferers' social lives. The outstanding feature of the study as a whole, and of the quote material in particular, is the broad range of areas of interaction with others that are affected. Thus, the work and social lives of sufferers are affected, throughout the life cycle, and sufferers engage in such tactics as avoidance of social situations and avoidance of particular activities within these situations, whilst adopting defensive manoeuvres. They are subjected to repeated verbal abuse, disgust and pity from others.

The rigour of Macgregor's (1951) approach to the subject group cannot be overlooked, since the project involved some 1400 interviews, with the time accruing to each subject ranging from 2 to 30 hours. Whilst an examination of the theoretical underpinnings of reliability and validity in qualitative studies is beyond the scope of this book, the coherence and consistency with which the picture of social disadvantage emerges from these interviews should itself serve to increase our confidence in the representativeness of these findings, at least with regard to the sample Macgregor investigates in such commendable depth. The final quote presented above indicates the degree to which sufferers' lives are apparently dominated by the need to adapt to social interactions. As Macgregor comments elsewhere (Macgregor 1990), it appears that disfigured people are denied the social anonymity that most of us enjoy in public situations.

In 1979, Macgregor published a follow-up study of 16 of the participants in the original 1951 study, examining their views following plastic surgery. Once again, the major content of the study is qualitative, and, indeed, Macgregor notes her belief that, whilst not 'representative' in the traditional sense required by quantitative scientific approaches current in medicine, the focusing of inquiry on to a few subjects who are examined in detail is more revealing than large-scale questionnaire studies which, by their nature, compress complex data into summary form. The superiority of in-depth interviews, for Macgregor, lies in their ability to elucidate personal elements of 'the human struggle and what it means to be visibly impaired'. Nevertheless, her approach is eclectic, and she does note that quantitative data from interviews with some 300 patients and relatives had been used to provide 'quantitative checks' on the qualitative data, although the process by which these checks were carried out is not described.

Seven full case histories are presented. In all these presentations, as well as in the isolated quotes in other parts of the text, the problematic nature of interactions with others forms the major strand of the respondents' narratives. Thus:

> I suffer tremendous fatigue, especially when I have to travel on subways. I have such anxiety facing people. I'm afraid of new people and I won't go anywhere.
>
> (Macgregor 1979: 13)

> I wanted to show her I was a human being – never mind the face.
>
> (Macgregor 1979: 21)

> The kids were making fun of me; I had no friends. … I built a wall around myself – maybe I didn't want to associate with them, but I thought they didn't want to associate with me….
>
> (Macgregor 1979: 35)

> When I'm introduced to the girl's parents, they smile sheepishly and seem at a loss for words.
>
> (Macgregor 1979: 44)

> I can't afford to get angry, because this attracts more attention.
>
> (Macgregor 1979: 45)

> It *never* leaves you. You're always self conscious about it….
>
> (Macgregor 1979: 61)

As in the earlier selections from Macgregor *et al.* (1953), not only is the breadth of the range of interactions affected clear, but the *preoccupation* of disfigured individuals with the reactions of others apparently accounts for the expenditure of much energy in social situations, as they are apparently both vigilant and prepared to react defensively to slights by others.

The notion of preoccupation with and preparation to respond to the reactions of others in social situations occurs in other first-hand accounts. James Partridge was severely burned in a car accident at age 18, and has spent a number of years campaigning on behalf of disfigured people. Partridge's account is not so much an autobiography as a series of suggestions for action for disfigured people, but is intimately based on his personal experiences. Thus, Partridge (1990) describes the 'SCARED' syndrome of social interactions between facially disfigured people and others. This model of social interaction with disfigured people is further described in Chapter 6, but is noted here since it is part of Partridge's description of his own experiences of coming into contact with others during the years following his own severe facial burns. He describes members of the public as exhibiting the following characteristic behaviours when coming into contact with disfigured people: staring, curiosity, awkwardness, rudeness, evasiveness, distance; whilst disfigured people themselves, according to Partridge, are submissive, clumsy, apathetic, regressive, excluded and defenceless. These personal notes, which became the core of Partridge's approach to treatment of social difficulties amongst disfigured people, present an often graphic account of his own difficulties, and more especially, his views of the reactions of others:

> Their eyes will feel like drills, adding psychological pain to your physical injuries. Even twenty years on, I do turn away from staring sometimes because of its intensity.
>
> (Partridge 1990: 90)

The impact of the behaviour of others on one's feelings is equally clear:

> The most frustrating thing about being stared at is that in only a few instances do you get the chance to explain that you are quite a normal person underneath.
>
> (Partridge 1990: 90)

In describing the curiosity which he has met in the eyes and words of others, Partridge offers an interesting first-hand description of behaviours which are entirely consistent with the novel stimulus hypothesis described earlier in this chapter:

> There will always be people who will blink hard at the sight of you, take a step backwards, avert their eyes, gasp, refuse to sit next to you, shield their children from you... None of these responses should surprise you ... they are part of the disfigured's lot.
>
> (Partridge 1990: 93)

The echoes of the novel stimulus hypothesis are particularly strong when he describes the way this curiosity interacts with anxiety and an embarrassed desire on the part of others not to stare, through the account of a personal friend's recollection of a first meeting with him:

> I'd have liked to have been able to look at you closely but was too self-conscious to do so – and too concerned as to what was the right course.

(Partridge 1990: 95)

Perhaps the most notable feature of Partridge's account, however, is the depth and sympathy with which he has examined the possible feelings of those who come into contact with disfigured people. He appears concerned not only with the ways in which non-disfigured people react to him, but with the anguish these people may themselves be undergoing. Nevertheless, it seems possible – from some of the other accounts, both by Partridge and by others, of the behaviours displayed towards disfigured people – that Partridge may be too kind in his ascription of positive motivations to non-disfigured people in their interactions with disfigured individuals. Descriptions of insulting behaviour towards disfigured people, whilst not systematically investigated, are common.

In the latter part of his book, and in his later writings (Partridge 1991, 1993; Partridge *et al.* 1994), Partridge has increasingly turned towards an examination of what may be done to help disfigured people, particularly in their social interactions with others. His approach to treatment is described in Chapter 6.

Christine Piff (1985) formed an influential self-help movement for facially disfigured people. Her approach, like Partridge's, focuses to a great extent on the social lives of sufferers, although 'Let's Face It' groups function much more as support and awareness-raising groups, rather than offering formal treatment in the way that Partridge now does. Piff writes movingly of her experience of disfigurement when her palate, eye socket, eye and much of one side of her face were removed for facial cancer in her 30s. Although Piff's experiences appear to be as much responses to being diagnosed with cancer and having to live with this life-threatening illness, her descriptions of her experiences are consistent with those of other disfigurement sufferers.

Piff's account presents graphic descriptions of the social difficulties faced by disfigured people. Perhaps the key element in her account is the range of situations affected. Thus, she found socialising difficult, but was also inhibited with her own family, whose possible reactions made her apprehensive, and was unable to return to her work as a nursery nurse. As in the various Macgregor accounts, a picture emerges of someone who spends considerable time monitoring the responses of others to her appearance.

Whilst health professionals are often praised in Piff's account, she is also aware of the shortcomings of the attempts by these clinicians to engage with the social difficulties of their patients. In an interview with Holmes (1986), she comments: 'I genuinely think most consultants involved with the facially disfigured think their patients cope beautifully'. This is perhaps overgenerous, since she recounts, in the same interview, a conversation with a young girl who describes how a ward sister, when asked how she might improve her looks after surgery for brain tumours, suggested, in front of a group of students, that she put a bucket over her head. Whilst it may be the case that health professionals are simply unaware of the emotional difficulties of disfigured people, it may also be that they deliberately avoid engaging with such emotions, because of the anxiety responses which they create in professionals themselves. Certainly, Bernstein (1976) has noted both the universality of such anxious responses to disfigured people, and the tendency of professionals to taunt disfigured children, which may likewise be a defensive reaction.

The formation of *Let's Face It* proved to be a significant turning point in Piff's adjustment to disfigurement. Bernstein (1976) describes a patient who coped with disfigurement by a process of self-objectification, involving allowing himself to be the subject of much experimentation, which might ultimately benefit other sufferers. As well as providing purpose, *Let's Face It* appears to have brought Piff into contact with many people, thus exposing her to potentially damaging or offensive reactions, which dangers she has overcome to create an influential nationwide network.

The selections in this section provide examples of the individual consequences of disfigurement which may underlie many of the group results provided by quantitative studies. Disfigured people are constantly under the scrutiny of others, and are restricted across the broad range of social situations. They are acutely aware of the responses of others and the generally negative attitudes these reveal. Social avoidance is a frequent consequence, and this can be either the total avoidance of social situations or withdrawal and lack of interaction within them. Disfigured people are constantly vigilant, and are denied the privacy of being ignored in social and public situations which non-disfigured individuals enjoy. As Partridge puts it:

> When you face the public, you will be scrutinised and automatic associations will be made in the public mind between your looks

and your character. These connections are rarely flattering, and will persist unless you challenge them.

(Partridge 1990: 123)

Exercise

Macgregor's (1990) 'social anonymity' is enjoyed by non-disfigured and non-disabled people to a considerable degree. Attempt to experience what happens when this anonymity is removed. Consider a tactic (wearing an eye patch, an arm bandage, unusually brightly coloured or soiled clothes, for example) to remove the anonymity you enjoy, then spend a morning shopping. Note the reactions of others. Some experiments have attempted to do just this, and are described in the next chapter.

Key further reading

Bull, R. and Rumsey, N. (1988) *The Social Psychology of Facial Appearance.* London: Springer-Verlag.
An excellent, detailed examination of facial attractiveness and disfigurement by two eminent psychological researchers in the field.

Goffman, E. (1963) *Stigma. Notes on the Management of Spoiled Identity.* Englewood Cliffs, New Jersey: Prentice-Hall.
A classic text.

Langer, E.J., Fiske, S., Taylor, S.E. and Chanowitz, B. (1976) Stigma, staring and discomfort: a novel stimulus hypothesis. *Journal of Experimental Social Psychology* 12, 451–63.
Reports the three studies by this group reported in this chapter. Worth reading in full.

Macgregor, F., Abel, T.M., Brut, A., Lauer, E. and Weissmann, S. (1953) *Facial Deformities and Plastic Surgery: A Psychosocial Study.* Springfield, Illinois: Thomas.
Superb account by the pre-eminent qualitative researcher in this field. Repays the effort involved in seeking it out.

Partridge, J. (1990) *Changing Faces: The Challenge of Facial Disfigurement.* London: Penguin.

Piff, C. (1985) *Let's Face It.* London: Victor Gollancz.
Two readable first-hand accounts by a burns survivor and a facial cancer survivor respectively.

Chapter 5

Disfigurement and social interaction

From the accounts presented in Chapter 4, we saw the range of difficulties experienced by disfigured people in social situations. This chapter explores these experiences in greater detail, but the focus here is on quantitative studies. These studies differ from subjective accounts and from qualitative studies in two major ways. First, they attempt to draw general trends from the data and argue that these trends are likely to be representative of the wider population of disfigured people. Second, they often attempt to draw out cause and effect relationships between the different variables being examined. In both these senses, such studies are potentially of great importance to clinical work, provided their methods are adequate to allow us to have confidence in their findings. This is because generalisability and the establishing of cause and effect relationships greatly increase the predictive value of the studies and in consequence permit us, to however imperfect a degree, to extrapolate from their findings to patients and clients we see in clinical practice. In other words, we can, to some extent, predict how they will be feeling and what they will do in response, following disfigurement, and this in turn can guide our assessments and interventions.

The social difficulties experienced by disfigured people are a major source of complaints by them, both in structured investigations by researchers and in the first-hand accounts written by disfigured individuals or recorded by such authors as Macgregor (e.g. Macgregor 1951) and Bernstein (1976) and reported in the previous chapter. Macgregor (1989) describes the key role of the face in regulating social interaction, including the importance of paralanguage and reliance by humans on the mediating effects of facial muscles on such communications as gaze and facial expression. In many cases of facial disfigurement (e.g. burns, palsy) such mediating movements are unavailable. Macgregor (1989) suggests that this leads to difficulty in 'reading' the faces of disfigured people, which in turn results in hesitancy and awkwardness. She sees disfigured people as consequently acutely aware of the reactions of others and as expending much energy in attention to the reactions of others, in preoccupation with appearance, and in 'defence mechanisms'. She concludes by suggesting that potentially fruitful areas of investigation include the effect of non-verbal communication on interactions with disfigured people and study of the extent to which the social distance experienced by disfigured people is a consequence of their appearance or their demeanour. Naturally, the face is not the only body part which mediates communication, although the social role of other body parts has been less studied in the disfigurement literature. We need only think for a moment of the role of the hands in mediating language, or the legs in mobility, to recognise the role of other parts of the body. Moreover, the body has a social role in presenting the self, and so it is likely that damage and disfigurement affecting any part of the body will have the potential to affect communication with others.

A number of studies exist which demonstrate that the stigmatisation recounted by disfigured people is generally observed in both laboratory and field situations, although the quality of such studies is variable. One fascinating account, whilst barely rising above the level of anecdote, gives an insight into the social world of the disfigured person. Carlisle (1991), a member of the staff of 'Nursing Times', donned make-up to simulate a scar and entered a variety of social situations. Whilst her account is certainly consistent with the accounts of many disfigured people, its chief relevance is to draw our attention to the possibility of bias in such studies. Although it would be strange if the repeated reports by disfigured people of stigmatising behaviour were all inaccurate, the Carlisle report reads as an object lesson in the inappropriate use of an assumed causative factor to explain observations. Thus, the presence of a scar is recounted by the author as a cause of both staring and looking away, and of both offering more and less help. Certainly, these differing responses might well both be generated by the presence of a scar, but considerable experimental control would be needed in order to exclude the effects of expectation on the part of the author. The need for caution in extrapolating from quantitative studies is just as great as it is when drawing inference from qualitative investigations. In fact, in some ways it is greater, since we are more accustomed to believing it is possible to generalise from the former. For this reason, the studies presented in the remainder of this chapter are examined with some critical analysis. Nevertheless, for reasons of space, complete coverage of the methodological aspects of even the small number of studies presented here is not possible, and the reader is directed to the original papers. The most important of these are noted in the key reading section.

Studies of social interactions with disfigured people

The strength of experimental and quasi-experimental studies lies in their attempts to exclude such bias from their examination of the difficulties faced by disfigured people. Kleck and Strenta (1980) showed that subjects believed reactions were being made to their simulated disfigurement even after this had been secretly removed. Twenty-four females interacted with confederates, having been led to believe that these confederates were also volunteers who had been informed subjects in one condition had epilepsy and in a second had an allergy. A third condition involved applying make-up to subjects to simulate the disfigurement. In fact, the confederates were unaware of the presumed status of the subjects and the simulated disfigurement had been removed via a subterfuge so that subjects in this group did not appear disfigured. Subjects in the epilepsy and disfigurement conditions reported significantly greater tenseness from confederates than allergy subjects, and disfigurement subjects made significantly greater reference to gaze behaviour. This study indicates possible difficulties in ascribing differences in people's behaviour to the presence of a stigma, but one major shortcoming of the experiment indicates that we should be cautious in extrapolating this conclusion to include genuinely disfigured or otherwise stigmatised people. The subject groups here did not, in fact, belong to such stigmatised groups. As a result, there is no reason to suppose that their perceptions and reactions would be similar to those of stigmatised people, unless it could be demonstrated that members of stigmatised groups shared the same expectancies of others' reactions to disfigurement as did non-members. A further distinction between the experimental group and stigmatised individuals is that the attention of the former has been drawn to the stigma as an active element of the experimental situation (in the case of the disfigured individual, involving considerable time and attention in the application of the disfigurement). It seems unlikely that this would not exert some influence on subject responses. In consequence, any generalisations to disfigured individuals from this study are extremely speculative. The difficulty in drawing conclusions from even carefully controlled experiments such as this indicates that anecdotal, journalistic accounts such as the Carlisle (1991) report do little to elucidate our knowledge of people's reactions to facial disfigurements.

Nevertheless, a body of research appears to offer objective support for the subjective experience of stigma described by disfigured people. It was suggested in the previous chapter that people avoid contact with disabled people because such individuals give rise to autonomic arousal and uncomfortable feelings of uncertainty (Kleck *et al.* 1966). Langer *et al.* (1976) suggested disabled people are avoided because they cause an unpleasant tension between the desire to stare at a novel stimulus and fear of offending the social prohibition against staring. Both these contentions seem relevant to an examination of reactions to disfigured people, whose 'disability' is highly visible. Worthington (1974) demonstrated that people choose greater interpersonal distance from an apparently disabled individual asking directions than from a control. Since the amount of personal space afforded the handicapped individual was greater, the author concluded that subjects were equally keen to help the stigmatised person (as shown by spending the same amount of time in contact), but did not want to catch whatever the person had. Although it is apparent that subjects reacted with avoidance to the stigmatised person, the study does not, in fact, clarify whether or not this was owing to fear of contamination, since less time spent with the individual might also be expected if such fear was the motivation behind offering greater personal space.

Building on Bernstein's (1976) observation that people tend to choose no closer than 'neutral' distance from disfigured people, Rumsey (1983) constructed an experiment to investigate such proxemic behaviour empirically, by observing the distance consecutive arrivals at a pedestrian crossing chose when standing next to a confederate waiting there, apparently with no visible facial defect, a birthmark, or scarring and bruising. Early arrivals stood significantly further from the confederate in both the birthmark and the scarring condition than the no disfigurement condition and further in the birthmark than in the scarring condition. Furthermore, first arrival subjects chose significantly more often to stand next to the non-disfigured side of the disfigured confederates.

This experiment suggests that subjects leave greater distance from disfigured individuals than from non-disfigured ones. Although it might be argued that there is a potential source of bias in reporting the distances involved, since the observers could never be truly blind to the conditions of the experiment, the index of stigmatising behaviour used (distance in centimetres) is sufficiently objective to allow us to be reasonably confident that this potential for bias had comparatively little effect on measurement. Moreover, although the choice of statistical test was suspect, an examination of the raw data renders such considerations almost redundant, since the differences in percentages of sides chosen were sufficiently large to render statistical treatment superfluous.

In a later study, Houston and Bull (1994) also investigated proxemic preferences of members of the public, by examining train seat occupancy in seats surrounding a confederate apparently with no visible defect, a birthmark, scarring or bruising. They found significantly less seat occupancy where the person appeared to have a birthmark than where no visible defect was simulated. Moreover, frequency of occupancy decreased the less normal the facial appearance became. Thus, no defect led to most occupancy, then bruising, then scarring, then birthmark. Taken together, these two experiments support the contention that disfigured people are avoided in public situations of minimal social interaction.

An early laboratory study by Kleck (1969) suggests that disabled people are also given greater social distance in more intimate settings. Twenty students were instructed in Origami (the Japanese art of paper folding) and required to teach it to a confederate either with or without a simulated leg amputation, ostensibly as part of a study of teaching. Apparent amputees were afforded significantly greater social distance on the first of two trials, but not the second. This is particularly interesting given that subjects also formed a *more positive* impression of the disabled than the non-disabled confederate during the first trial, but not the second. The authors suggest that this formation of a more positive impression of the disabled confederate may conform to our tendency in society to be kind to disadvantaged individuals. Moreover, the finding of increased proximity on the second trial is consistent with the findings of Langer *et al.* (1976) and with the interpretation of these findings in conditioning terms offered in Chapter 4. It is possible to speculate that the initial favourable evaluation of the disabled confederate is itself a defence against anxiety, and, like social avoidance, decreases on subsequent exposure because anxiety reduces. This in turn leads to the speculation that our norm of kindness to disadvantaged individuals is, in general, an anxiety-based response. Certainly, the tendency to 'kindness' was not translated into action, in terms of physical proximity, in the Kleck (1969) study. Indeed, it seemed to be inversely related to it: the more positive your impression of the disabled person, the further away from them you sit! Koster and Bergsma (1990) note that 'positive' reactions such as sympathy and pity are displayed to disfigured people. However, it is over-simple to assume that such displays are positive. The supposed tendency to kindness may, indeed, be little more than an aspect of establishing our dissimilarity from the disabled person, and an aspect of stigma, or indeed of anxiety reduction via cognitive avoidance through the establishing of that differentness, with consequent lessening of the fear that what has befallen the disfigured individual might happen to ourselves. Certainly, disfigured individuals report resenting both the pity of others (Andreason and Norris 1972) and their *unkind behaviour* (see Chapter 4).

The above studies together support the notion that disfigured individuals are indeed stigmatised in public social situations, at least if we regard avoidance of contact as an indicator of stigmatisation. It should be noted, however, that these studies involved relatively superficial contact. There are no field studies which directly demonstrate avoidance of disfigured people in situations where more intimate social interaction is present, although anecdotal accounts are frequent (see Chapter 4). However, studies of attractiveness in more intimate situations generally favour more attractive individuals, and disfigured people are often rated at the low end of the attractiveness continuum. For a review of this literature, readers may wish to examine Rumsey (1983), Bull and Rumsey (1988) or Newell (1998).

Kleck *et al.* (1966) suggested that the behavioural repertoire displayed with disabled people will be stereotyped, inhibited and over-controlled. They examined these assertions in two laboratory studies, in which an interviewer appeared either disabled or able-bodied. As in many such studies, it is impossible to tease out the different possible contributions made by impairment of function and appearance. In the first experiment, the study was presented to fifty-six undergraduates as an opinion survey. Contrary to expectations, subjects talked for longer and reported liking the interviewer more in the disabled condition, although the same confederate took both roles. There was, however, less variation in answers to questions in the disabled condition, suggesting more over-control of responses. There were two methodological difficulties, noted by the authors, which led them to discount the results of this first experiment. The behaviour of the confederate was not consistent across the conditions, and there was the possibility that desire to help a disabled person may have caused the longer answers in the disabled condition. Since there is a correlation between length of answers to open questions and perception of positiveness of the interview by interviewees, this might have influenced interviewee liking of the interviewer. Moreover, the authors wished to make the disability of the interviewer more obvious.

The second experiment was generally similar to the first, but with less emphasis placed on verbal behaviour in explanations to subjects, less information regarding the interviewer's adjustment to disability and a more visible disability (apparent amputee). Subjects who interacted with the disabled confederate were also subsequently divided by the researchers into groups who did (H+) or did not (H−) express subjective discomfort in the presence of the handicapped interviewer.

Psycho-galvanic skin response of the forty-six subjects was measured and was significantly different between the disabled and non-disabled conditions in both H+ and H− groups. Thus, both those who expressed discomfort and those who did not were equally physiologically aroused in the presence of the disabled confederate.

Those in the disabled group took significantly longer to complete a question selection task than those in the non-disabled group, and terminated the interview sooner. This latter feature was more marked in the H+ group. Visual inspection of data suggested that the H+ group showed less variance in their responses than the H− group, who in turn showed less than subjects in the non-disabled condition, indicating greater over-control of their behaviours. Finally, H+ subjects showed more distortion of their expressed opinions from those later reported outside the experimental situation than did H− subjects, who showed less than those in the non-disabled condition, suggesting greatest desire to make the disabled person feel comfortable on the part of H+ subjects.

The authors note that definition of subgroups (H+ and H−) for comparisons after selection for inclusion in the study was problematic, because some other variable, such as personality, may have led to the differences in their scores, but suggest that this is mitigated by the fact that the H+ subgroup results confirm rather than contradict trends in other areas of the data. This is possibly an inadequate justification for this methodological difficulty. It might reasonably be expected that anxious people would behave in this way regardless of condition, and no attempt was made to isolate an uncomfortable group from subjects in the *non-disabled* condition. Moreover, the authors do not report whether subjects said they were uncomfortable *because* of the handicap of the interviewer. Finally, H+ were not more physiologically aroused than H−, so that the observed differences might simply be a consequence of differences between individuals who do or do not admit to discomfort, rather than between those who are or are not uncomfortable.

This makes it extremely difficult to draw any conclusions as to whether or not level of discomfort affects level of interaction with a disabled person. The H+ group did, however, report less previous experience of disabled people, which makes a valid prospective distinction between the two groups possible, on the basis of this past exposure rather than discomfort. The work of Langer *et al.* (1976) is relevant here. Their paper was described in Chapter 4 because of its relevance to their novel stimulus hypothesis of people's reactions to disabled individuals. The third experiment involved face-to-face interaction with an apparently disabled person, and prior visual exposure resulted in a diminution of the difference between interpersonal distances in the disabled and non-disabled groups to non-significant levels. If we accept the novel stimulus hypothesis, the differences between the behaviours of H+ and H– subjects in the Kleck *et al.* (1966) experiment may have been caused by lack of previous exposure to disabled individuals. However, this past exposure did not lead the behaviour of the H– group to resemble that of subjects in the non-disabled group. The effect of prior exposure seems modest in the Kleck *et al.* (1966) experiment.

Despite methodological difficulties, the Kleck *et al.* (1966) investigation is an important study, which suggests people behave differently in the presence of disabled individuals, showing more over-controlled behaviour and seeking to avoid contact, whilst also having a desire to help by setting the person at ease through expressing similar opinions. It is unfortunate that this potentially fruitful line of investigation has not really been explored in the many years following this study.

The general picture provided by the above studies of social interactions with disfigured people supports anecdotal reports of their stigmatisation by others, and the evidence that disfigured people mistakenly attribute the behaviours of others to their own disfigurements is slight. Bernstein's (1976) contention that disfigured people are afforded greater social distance by others is supported by studies of proxemic behaviour both in public situations and in more private one-to-one encounters. The repertoire of behaviours exhibited in the presence of disfigured people may be reduced and over-controlled. However, the possible mechanisms which might underlie these behaviours have not, as yet, been satisfactorily investigated, although it seems probable that anxiety might play a part in responses to disfigured people. Similarly the effect of previous contact with disfigured people, which may be related to level of anxiety, requires further examination. We have little information as to how far facial disfigurement hinders disfigured people in more intimate social circumstances.

Helping behaviour

Helping behaviour has received considerable study in the literature concerning disability and disfigurement, and an understanding of the conditions under which disfigured people are or are not helped might both elucidate the motivations involved in helping and aid in developing ways of altering public attitudes to disfigured people and interactions with them.

The possibly contradictory elements of desire to terminate contact and desire to help a stigmatised person were investigated by Doob and Ecker (1970) in a study which offered 121 housewife subjects the choice of returning a questionnaire through the post or completing it in an interview by a confederate either wearing or not wearing an eye patch. In the interview condition, there was no difference between the disfigured/ non-disfigured groups, but in the postal return condition more subjects both accepted and returned the questionnaire in the disfigured group, a finding the authors conclude indicates that subjects are likely to offer *more* help to a disfigured person, providing no additional contact is required. The concomitant conclusion is that the competing desires to be helpful and to avoid contact cancel each other out in the interview condition, where additional contact is required. By contrast, Soble and Strickland (1974) found that confederates who appeared to have a hunchback were less likely to gain agreement from doorstep solicitation for an interview at a later date with themselves than control confederates. In this study, it appears that desire to end contact was mediated not by any greater willingness to help the stigmatised person, but merely by desire to avoid contact on both the current and subsequent occasions.

The possibility that disfigured individuals might be no more likely to be helped in situations where contact was required was further investigated by Samerotte and Harris (1976), who also examined the role of perceived responsibility and requesting help in determining the likelihood of help being offered. One hundred and twenty subjects were exposed to a confederate dropping envelopes in a shopping centre. The confederate was either a non-disabled control, or had an arm bandage or an eye patch and facial scar. In each of these three conditions, the confederate either did or did not blame subjects for causing the envelopes to be dropped and did or did not request help. Although requests for help did not affect compliance, subjects were more likely to help the bandaged confederate than either the disfigured or control confederates (who received equal help), and were more likely to help if blamed for causing the envelopes to be dropped.

The authors suggest that the tendency to avoid a disfigured person may have counteracted any increased sympathy felt for them. However, although the researchers were careful to ensure that the arm bandage did not interfere with ability to pick up the envelopes, it could nevertheless have led to a perception of more difficulty in so doing, since a bandaged arm might reasonably be supposed by subjects to indicate weakness or impairment of this area. By contrast, the disfigured confederate might not have been assumed to be handicapped in the task by lacking the sight of an eye. Rather than being counteracted by a desire for avoidance, neither desire for avoidance nor increased sympathy for the disfigured confederate need have been present. The disfigured confederate, unlike the bandaged confederate, may simply have been perceived as being as able to perform the task as the control. However, despite this methodological difficulty, the study does offer a further demonstration that disfigured people receive *no more* help than non-disfigured, even if the motivation for this is not adequately investigated.

Levitt and Kornhaber (1977), in a study of handicap not related specifically to the face, attempted to examine whether a non-stigmatising handicap would produce as much compliance as a stigmatising one. The stigmatising handicap was wearing leg braces and half crutches, to denote a permanent handicap, rather than a plaster cast and wooden crutches to denote a temporary and, it is argued, non-stigmatising incapacity. A control confederate was also used. The confederates approached 60 male and 60 female pedestrians and asked for spare change. Significantly more people gave money to both handicapped confederates than to controls, but there was no difference between the stigmatised and non-stigmatised confederates. However, significantly more *money* was given to the non-stigmatised than the control confederate, although there was no significant difference either between the stigmatised and non-stigmatised or between the stigmatised and control confederates. The paper offers some support for the contention that both stigmatised and non-stigmatised handicapped individuals are likely to receive more help than controls, but it should be noted that the degree of interaction required for helping was minimal.

In another, better-conducted, study which again involved face-to-face contact, but with slightly more interaction, Shaw *et al.* (1980) investigated frequency of petition signing in response to male and female petitioners with or without a facial disfigurement (burn scar, birthmark or protruding teeth), dividing the petition condition itself into contentious and non-contentious issues. They approached 7200 potential signatories, to explore the hypothesis that disfigured individuals would be more avoided and get fewer signatures, and divided subject response into a five-point scale, from evasion (no acknowledgement of the confederate) through polite refusal, reasoned refusal, hostile refusal, to signing.

Contrary to expectations, there was no significant effect of disfigurement on evasion, although controls obtained significantly more signatures than did disfigured confederates in the uncontentious petition condition. There was no such effect in the contentious petition. The authors suggest that the uncontentious petition maximised the salience of the disfigurement cue. They account for lack of avoidance of disfigured individuals by suggesting that this may have resulted from a suspension of the ban on staring, allowing them to indulge their desire to look. However, subjects might equally well have responded to a general tendency to comply at least to the extent of polite refusal (which might even, as the authors suggest, have been enhanced by desire to appear sympathetic to a stigmatised person). Alternatively, the desire to avoid disfigured people might be apparent only in situations where there is considerable anxiety. This anxiety might be aroused only in situations of interaction more intimate than passing on the street.

Piliavin *et al.* (1975) suggested a two stage model of helping behaviour which asserted that emergency situations exert on bystanders a desire to decrease arousal felt in the presence of such situations. The particular circumstances of the emergency will combine with personality characteristics of the bystander to influence either rapid helping or escape. The bystander will respond so as to reduce arousal as rapidly as possible and incur as few other costs as possible. Costs may be incurred by helping (e.g. danger, exposure to revolting experiences) or not helping (e.g. continued arousal, self-blame, blame from others). These two stages of arousal and calculation of profit and loss are seen as an alternative to the notion that helping is mediated simply by greater liking. Liking and attractiveness of the helped person are merely elements of the profit and loss equation in the Piliavin *et al.* (1975) account.

This model has considerable explanatory power in considering the responses of individuals to facially disfigured people, who may be associated both with greater loss in the equation, if their appearance gives rise to greater arousal in the potential helper, and with less profit, if they are perceived as unattractive, or if their good opinion of the helper is otherwise perceived as not valuable. Piliavin *et al.* (1975) investigated the relevance of the two stage model to helping behaviour with facially disfigured individuals in an experiment which sought to isolate the effect of stigmatisation in reducing helping behaviour from the possible effects of perceived worthlessness of or danger from the helpee. In their study, a confederate either with or without a 'large, red birthmark' (a feature construed by the authors as unrelated to either character of the victim or potential danger of the crisis to the helper), apparently fell in a subway train, and the frequency of helping behaviours was recorded. The unmarked victim was helped on 86.4% of trials, whilst the marked individual was helped on 60.7%, a highly significant difference, indicating clear support for the notion that facial disfigurement constitutes a cost in helping situations.

In an attempt to account for findings such as Doob and Ecker's (1970) in terms of the Piliavin *et al.* (1975) model, Ungar (1979) examined the amount that a confederate with a medical eye patch was helped by passers-by following inaccurate directions received from a further confederate. The author predicted that the stimulus person with the eye patch would be helped less than a control *only* under a high effort condition. Under this condition, passers-by seeking to correct the incorrect directions had to follow the confederate along a subway platform. In the low effort condition, the confederate remained standing next to the chosen passer-by. It was found that the eye patch confederate was helped less in the high effort condition. The author concluded that this stigma led subjects to attend more to the additional cost involved in the high effort condition. However, it might equally well be suggested, from the results, that contact with an individual bearing a stigma itself constitutes a cost (as seems apparent from, for example, Piliavin *et al.* 1975; Rumsey 1983; Houston and Bull 1994), which, when added to the cost involved in spending time following the individual, is sufficient to inhibit helping behaviour. No concept of increased sensitivity to already existing costs is necessary; the stigma constitutes an additional cost.

In Bull and Stevens' (1981) study of helping behaviour in collecting for charity, they suggest that expected duration of contact is likely to be an important aspect of such behaviour. However, it should also be noted that duration should be expected to interact with other indices of intimacy, such as spatial proximity. The authors studied the interactions of a confederate either with or without a simulated port wine stain with subjects from whom they collected money door-to-door for a children's charity. There was what the authors describe as an 'almost significant' ($P < 0.10$) effect of disfigurement on amount of money donated, with more money donated to non-disfigured than disfigured. It is interesting to note, given the suggestion in the literature that social skills training might be a useful component in helping disfigured people cope with negative interactions with others, that there was no interaction between disfigurement and gaze, nor any main effect of gaze on contribution. The authors suggest that their data support the notion that facial disfigurement may lead to less helping behaviour.

In a series of three experiments which examined levels of helping behaviour at different levels of interaction, Rumsey (1983) first undertook a partial replication of Benson *et al.*'s (1976) study of helping of more and less attractive individuals by retrieval of lost application forms (including photographs of the applicants) from telephone booths, on this occasion comparing non-disfigured photographs with those of individuals with either a birthmark or trauma scarring. As in the original Benson *et al.* (1976) study, the number of applications forwarded was the index of helping behaviour. Rumsey (1983) found no significant effect of disfigurement on helping behaviour, although she does note that some subjects may have been more motivated to help the confederate's father, who was presented as having been responsible for leaving the application, rather than the confederate. However, it should be noted that this did not appear to have been the case in the Benson *et al.* (1976) study, which *did* find significant differences between the help received by attractive and unattractive confederates. Other aspects of Rumsey's (1983) discussion of the non-significant finding are illuminating from a methodological standpoint, since she notes that sympathy for a disfigured person might have outweighed bias against them, and balanced the desire to help the more attractive non-disfigured target person. She also suggests that, in the privacy of the booth, the suspension of the norm against staring may have led subjects to attend more closely to the information about the disfigured person, and thus increase the likelihood of their returning the form. It should be noted that, as in the Benson *et al.* study, no interaction is required in Rumsey's first study, and so generalisations from it to more intimate forms of helping should be modest.

In the second experiment in Rumsey (1983), a minimal level of interaction was introduced, as disfigured (birthmark) and non-disfigured confederates collected in the street for a children's charity. She points out that no social interaction was necessary in order to contribute. The level of interaction was thus marginally lower than either the Bull and Stevens (1981) or Shaw *et al.* (1980) studies. Subjects were passers-by, whose numbers were counted by discreet observation. There was no difference in the percentage of individuals helping nor in the amount of money donated in each condition, although there was a general tendency for more people in the non-disfigured condition to be helped, but for more money to be given by those who did help in the disfigured condition. These results are, therefore, generally similar to those of Bull and Stevens (1981), who likewise found no effect of disfigurement on helping.

In the final study, Rumsey (1983) had a disfigured (birthmark) or non-disfigured confederate solicit respondents for a survey on television viewing and current affairs. The potential level of interaction in this study was, therefore, greater than in Bull and Stevens' (1981) and perhaps as great as in other mock survey studies (Doob and Ecker 1970; Soble and Strickland 1974). Rumsey (1983) cites the former of these studies as an example of disfigured individuals receiving more help, although it should be noted that this was the case only in the postal questionnaire return element of this study. In the element requiring continuing face-to-face interaction, and thus most similar to Rumsey's third study, no difference was found between the conditions. In Rumsey's own study, although there was a marked tendency for disfigured people to be helped less, this did not reach significance. Once again, there is no unequivocal evidence from this study that disfigured individuals are helped more or less than non-disfigured persons. Nevertheless, it should be noted again that the level of interaction in the final study was still fairly small when compared with most social interactions.

Although it has been suggested (Rumsey 1983) that, under certain circumstances, disfigured people might be afforded more help than their non-disfigured counterparts, the evidence for this is slight. Of the studies here, those which require any major level of personal contact suggest that the disfigured person is afforded no advantage (Doob and Ecker 1970; Bull and Stevens 1981; Rumsey 1983) or is discriminated against (Soble and Strickland 1974; Piliavin *et al.* 1975; Levitt and Kornhaber 1977; Ungar 1979).

Moreover, it appears that desire to avoid contact with disfigured people, rather than simply cancelling out some proportion of the amount of desire to help, often eliminates that desire completely. It also seems, from the Piliavin *et al.* (1975) study, that this desire is mediated by revulsion caused by the disfigurement, rather than by either derogation of presumed personality characteristics, or perceived dangerousness of the disfigured person (although the first contention should be treated with caution, given the tendency to derogate less attractive individuals and the likelihood that a disfigured person will be viewed as unattractive). It is interesting to note that this experiment required considerably more close contact with confederates than did investigations of helping behaviour which found little or no negative effect or found a positive effect of disfigurement on helping. It may be the case that disfigured people enjoy the same or better social responses compared with other members of the population only in conditions where minimal contact is required. This is congruent with Bernstein's (1976) assertion of the preference for neutral social distance in interacting with disfigured people.

Judgements of social competence of disfigured people

The subjective accounts of disfigured people of their experiences in social interactions have been summarised in Chapter 4. It has also been noted that some commentators have cast doubt on the accuracy of disfigured people's perceptions of the reactions of others to them (e.g. Kleck and Strenta 1980; Shaw 1986). Rumsey *et al.* (1986b) explored the effect of the behaviour of facially disfigured people on the reactions of others in a videotaped study of a confederate with or without a port wine stain who demonstrated either good or bad social skills with 12 female subjects. The socially competent confederate was rated as more warm and friendly by subjects and as more warm, friendly, likeable, interesting and competent by independent observers. Moreover, subjects smiled more and showed lower response latencies towards the socially competent confederate. These findings were *not* influenced by whether the confederate was facially disfigured. Rumsey *et al.* conclude that social skill might exert sufficient influence to override the negative influence of stigmatisation as a result of facial disfigurement, and suggest the use of a social skills training programme to help disfigured people in learning to be active in overcoming such stigmatisation.

This suggestion receives tangential support from the finding that social skill is possibly interactively linked with attractiveness. Attractive people are generally perceived as more socially skilled. Moreover, people who are *believed* by subjects to be attractive are rated as more socially skilled, sight unseen, by independent raters, than people believed to be unattractive. This appears to be a response to confirmatory behaviour elicited by those who interact with the target individuals believing them to be attractive or unattractive (Snyder *et al.* 1977). Furthermore, attractive individuals actually do display greater social skill, even when they are unseen by those with whom they interact (Goldman and Lewis 1977). Goldman and Lewis had independent observers rate the attractiveness of sixty male and sixty female participants engaged in 5-minute telephone conversations with each other, whilst subjects rated their partners for social skill and according to their desire to interact with them again in the future. There was high inter-rater reliability for measurement of attractiveness of the subjects, and these ratings were positively correlated with ratings of their social skills by the other subjects with whom they interacted ($r = 0.31$ males, $r = 0.29$ females). Although these correlations are low, the authors note that this could have been caused by the naturalistic way in which the interactions were allowed to progress. In any event, the study offers some support for the contention that attractiveness may be genuinely associated with greater social skill, possibly as a result of greater opportunities for successful social interaction experienced by attractive people in early life. On this basis, it may be argued that those who come into contact with attractive people believe they are likely to be socially skilled at least partly on the basis of previous interactions with attractive, socially skilled people, and believe the reverse of unattractive people with whom they interact. In consequence, they encourage both attractive and unattractive people to exhibit behaviours consistent with either their stereotypes or genuine previous experiences of such people. Extrapolating this finding to disfigured people, it is possible to argue that an enhancement of their social skills may be necessary in two ways: to counteract the negative expectations of others and, for those who have been disfigured for a considerable time, to improve upon the impoverished social skills they actually possess as a result of previous exposure to non-rewarding social interactions with those who expect them to be socially unskilled or unrewarding and thus elicit such unskilled behaviours from them.

The notion that judgements of attraction are subject to influence from judgements of social competence receives further support from Bull and Brooking's (1986) study, in which sixty psychology undergraduates were shown photographs of interview participants and were asked to evaluate them. Stimulus photographs were represented to subjects as either married or unmarried and were edited to look physically disfigured on 50% of occasions. Stimulus people were thus paired with either a married or unmarried partner (the titles Miss and Mrs being used to distinguish between conditions), with either the male or female partner appearing disfigured. The male disfigured participant was judged to be significantly more intelligent and attractive when married (to a non-disfigured partner). Females were judged to be significantly less likeable when the male partner was disfigured, whether married to him or not. However, when females were represented as married to a non-disfigured male, the fact that the females themselves were or were not disfigured had no effect on judgements of their attractiveness. When unmarried, they were judged significantly less attractive when disfigured. There were no conditions in which both males and females had a disfigurement. The authors conclude that facial disfigurement does not influence judgements of attractiveness if you are married, and that this may mean that judgements of the disfigured may be influenced by their achievements and skills. This in turn may mean that, through such achievements, they may be able to overcome society's prejudice against them. This last suggestion is perhaps over-optimistic. Although the authors do not say so, their suggestion appears to be related to the contention in Sigall and Landy (1973) that we may impute positive characteristics to people associated with attractive partners. This possibility is also implied by Bar-Tal and Saxe (1976). However, the evidence from these studies is equivocal and is restricted to relatively narrowly focused experimental situations which may lack external validity, although the Bull and Brooking (1986) study overcame several impediments to external validity. It *may* be that disfigurement made no difference to attractiveness judgements of disfigured people in the presence of non-disfigured partners because they were assumed to have positive qualities which compensated for their disfigurement, but there is no direct evidence for this in the Bull and Brooking (1986) study, since such assumptions were not tested.

Social skill may influence stigmatising judgements applied to disfigured people by others, although investigation of the role of social skill in this context is at an early stage. Moreover, given the possibility that disfigured people, like unattractive individuals, may be perceived as less socially skilled than others, the disfigured person may require training in social performance in order to offset this perception. The fact that disfigured people may, in fact, have less opportunity to practice and receive reinforcement for appropriate socially skilled performance potentially increases the need for such training, although this last contention is speculative and itself requires further examination. Although the suggestion that achievement may enable disfigured people to overcome society's prejudice is intriguing, it requires much more investigation.

The studies presented in this chapter increase the amount of credence we can give to the general applicability of qualitative insights into the difficulties of disfigured people, and the accounts of disfigured people themselves. There is, however, considerable variability in the quality of the studies, and the overall volume of work in this area remains small. Indeed, apart from small pockets of activity (in particular by Rumsey, Bull and their various collaborators) there appears to be no sustained effort to investigate the plight of disfigured individuals in their social lives. Nevertheless, some trends emerge. It is likely that disfigured people experience stigma from others, and that this response is mediated by anxiety on the part of such others. It is likely that such stigmatisation is in response to the disfigurement rather than to other qualities of the disfigured person, although social skill may offset this to some degree. Moreover, the contention that this may be offset, in certain circumstances, by the desire to help disfigured people receives little support. In the following chapter, we shall explore the psychological difficulties experienced by disfigured people and examine some attempts to address these difficulties.

Key further reading

Benson, P.L., Karabenick, S.A. and Lerner, R.M. (1976) Pretty Pleases: the effects of physical attractiveness, race and sex on receiving help. *Journal of Experimental Social Psychology* 12, 409–15.

Bernstein, N.R. (1982) Psychological results of burns. The damaged self-image. *Clinics in Plastic Surgery* 9(3), 337–46.

Houston, V. and Bull, R. (1994) Do people avoid sitting next to someone who is facially disfigured? *European Journal of Social Psychology* 24, 279–84.

Rumsey, N. (1983) *Psychological problems associate with facial disfigurement.* Unpublished PhD thesis, North East London Polytechnic.

Samerotte, G.C. and Harris, M.B. (1976) Some factors influencing helping: the effects of a handicap, responsibility and requesting help. *Journal of Social Psychology* 98, 39–45.

Chapter 6

Psychosocial disturbance in disfigurement, and its treatment

The nature and extent of psychosocial disturbance

Accurate estimation of the prevalence and individual level of psychological disturbance amongst disfigured people is hampered by a number of difficulties within the literature. Martin *et al.* (1988) provided only a general index of handicap from their comprehensive sample, without providing specific measures of any domains of disturbance (e.g. physical, social, psychological). Studies which have focused more precisely on types of difficulty have, by contrast, used samples drawn from particular patient subpopulations (e.g. burns survivors, port wine stain sufferers). Whilst these studies have offered more detailed information regarding patterns of difficulty, they are typically of small numbers of participants. Moreover, they cannot, alone, allow the drawing of any general conclusions about the effects of disfigurement, since these effects are likely to be mediated by differing factors amongst the different participant groups. General conclusions about psychological difficulties faced by disfigured people must therefore arise from a synthesis of the studies of these different subpopulations.

In an early and much-quoted study, Andreason and co-workers examined adaptation mechanisms (Andreason and Norris 1972) and psychiatric morbidity (Andreason *et al.* 1971) in 20 patients following severe burn injuries. The findings of Andreason and Norris (1972) suggest that a majority of patients adjust well, despite the difficulty of the task involved. Of particular note is their use of the expression 'progressive desensitisation' to describe the process whereby patients become accustomed to their appearance, overcoming anxiety when faced with the changed appearance. Although not described precisely in the terms used by Wolpe (1958) in his formulation of systematic desensitisation as a treatment for phobic disorders, it is clear from the context that Andreason and Norris have in mind the process of overcoming anxiety through repeated exposure, in a way similar to that explored in this book.

In a paper focusing particularly on the psychiatric profiles of the subjects in Andreason and Norris (1972), Andreason *et al.* (1971) attempted to examine the incidence and types of psychiatric complications arising and to determine whether these problems were predictable. The paper consists of a number of case histories and a table of pathological and demographic characteristics of the participants. Of their sample, five individuals had psychiatric problems which pre-dated their burn, whilst a further five had acquired psychiatric diagnoses subsequently. Unfortunately the report does not make clear which diagnoses pre-dated and post-dated the burns. The occurrence of psychiatric complications following burns, even in the study sample, is thus uncertain, and the issue is further complicated by the description of only six of these individuals as having current emotional problems. In general, however, they conclude a generally optimistic prognosis for burns victims, with comparatively mild psychological discomfort amongst affected individuals. Once again, the numbers involved are too small to permit definitive conclusions. Whilst important because they represent early attempts to follow up burns-disfigured people in a systematic way, the findings should be treated with care because of the low numbers involved and the tendency of the authors to make generalised assertions based on these small numbers.

Malt's (1980) review of follow-up studies of burns patients concluded that the overall incidence of psychosocial difficulties amongst burned adults was unlikely to be less than 30% in an unselected group. Their difficulties were likely to comprise anxiety syndromes, reduced social interaction without specific mental illness, and possible organic psychosyndromes. Furthermore, the rate and severity of problems was likely to increase with level of severity of disability. However, Malt also noted that the seven long-term follow-ups he was able to identify contained numerous methodological flaws. Most were of small numbers, obtained small participation rates from the parent populations, and often investigated only more serious burns. Demographic descriptions were inadequate and the use of different methods made it difficult to draw conclusions across studies, with no consistency in the definition of problems. No comparisons of rates of disturbance with the general population were undertaken. The study groups were not divided into adults and children, or by aetiology of the burn. Taken together, these problems limited the conclusions that Malt was able to draw from the studies reviewed.

In a later empirical study, Malt and Ugland (1989) addressed some of these shortcomings. They examined a group of 70 (57 males, 13 females) burned adults at between 3 and 13 years post injury. The majority of the group had sustained minor injuries. At follow-up, 23% suffered definite psychosocial adjustment problems sufficient to interfere with life in a significant way, and patients with more severe injuries had a higher rate of disturbance (44%) than those with minor injuries (16%). None of those rated as severe were working (11.4%). The authors noted that their overall rate of 23% corresponded well with a US study (Blumenfield and Reddish 1987). The source of the disturbance, whether from disfigurement, physical impairment or post-traumatic reaction, is not, however, investigated.

In a smaller study of a clinical group, Faber *et al.* (1987) screened 42 burned adults for psychological and social problems and followed them up, finding that 21% needed psychological help at 18 months post injury. Their study is somewhat supported by Wallace's (1988) findings of psychosocial disturbance in a group of forty-five discharged burns patients 6 months after discharge and a further forty at 2 years post discharge. The Wallace study, although once again small, is strengthened by the use of discharged patients, since there is possible bias in studies of patients currently attending, for example, plastic surgery outpatients (Rumsey 1983). One might expect that current attenders would differ from discharged patients in a number of ways. They might be hopeful, since treatment was still in progress and they might continue to have possibly unrealistic expectations about the possible benefits of treatment . They might also be in a state of denial of their difficulties as part of grieving over their lost appearance (Bernstein 1976). Conversely, their ratings might be high because of the effect of undergoing treatment. The use of a post-discharge group reduces this source of variability.

At 2 years post discharge, 30–40% of adults in the Wallace study showed severe psychological difficulties, whilst 75% of children aged under 1 year when burned showed severe emotional and behavioural disturbance. In spite of this, *none* were receiving professional help related to their psychological difficulties, and over half relied on fellow patients as sources of support. Furthermore, although half were in regular contact with health professionals at 6 months and 40% at 2 years post discharge, less than 25% felt they had *any* useful contact with any professional related to their burns. At 6 months, all patients would have valued some form of help, including staff-led talks, individual professional help, newsletters and self-help groups. This picture was generally confirmed at 2 years.

In a similar survey of ex-patients at 1 year follow-up, Williams and Griffiths (1991) found that practical advice, information and emotional support were the most wanted interventions. Most significantly, 30% of respondents reported wanting intervention prior to discharge, 30% at discharge and a mere 4% at 6 months after discharge, indicating that respondents would greatly value timely interventions regarding potential sources of post-burns difficulties.

As in the Faber *et al.* (1987) study, the site of the burn is not identified by Wallace (1988), although the inference from her paper is that disfigurement is a major issue for respondents. Although numbers in both the Wallace (1988) and Williams and Griffiths (1991) studies were small, and further reduced on many of the specific questions by incomplete responses, the sheer size of the discrepancies reported between the perceived need of respondents and responses to that need should give professionals working in the area considerable pause.

In a study of people with port wine stains, Kalick *et al.* (1981) suggested that the level of distress described by sufferers is sometimes out of proportion to the extent of the disfigurement, although they do not cite any evidence for this assertion. Kalick *et al.*'s study showed sufferers did not differ from normative groups on a number of scales for which normative data exist, measuring introversion, neuroticism, anxiety and depression. Indeed, of the battery of tests they gave, only one anxiety subscale differed from such normative data. However, 43 of the eventual 79 respondents reported that their port wine stain had affected the way in which others treated them.

The authors suggested several reasons for the lack of correspondence between their study findings and those of several earlier papers. The kinds of individuals attending clinics since the earlier studies might have changed, the interviewing in these earlier studies might have been biased, or the measures of their own study too insensitive. Finally, it was considered possible that port wine stain patients were more resilient than other disfigured individuals, partly because of a high level of family support. These suggestions are, however, largely without basis. Neither of the two studies they mention (Edgerton *et al.* 1961; Reich 1969) was of port wine stain patients, so suppositions about the role of changing clinic attenders over the years are irrelevant. The two types of sample are simply different, regardless of time. Speculation about differences in the adequacy of the measurement approaches applied across the studies are likewise rendered impossible by the differences between the sample groups. The differences found might, as the authors suggest, lead us to suppose that port wine stain patients are more resilient than others, but, since no measure of *level* of disfigurement was made in any of the studies, this, rather than *cause* of the disfigurement, might have led to score differences. The authors' rationale for suggesting greater family support is extremely limited, being supported only by the anecdotal noting, by the authors, that port wine stain patients were invariably accompanied to the outpatients' clinic by family members.

The possible difficulty of using questionnaires to investigate psychological adjustment is highlighted in a study of patients with port wine stains by Lanigan and Cotterill (1989). They followed the assertion by Kalick *et al.* (1981) that psychological disturbance may be missed by insensitive tests, and reported a discrepancy between two standardised measures of minor psychological morbidity (General Health Questionnaire (GHQ) and Hospital Anxiety and Depression (HAD)) and their own twenty-six dichotomous question instrument. Considerable numbers of their seventy-one respondents reported difficulties, stating, for example, they would feel better about themselves if their birthmarks were improved by treatment, more comfortable with the opposite sex, and with the same sex. Respondents also believed that people stared at them because of their birthmarks, and that it had affected their self-confidence, and reported the need to hide the mark. These suggestions of disturbance were in contrast to the small numbers of positive scores on the HAD and GHQ.

The authors conclude that their study represents a further instance in which the use of questionnaires aimed at specific areas of disturbance in port wine stain individuals reveals such difficulties, whilst these are not detectable on standardised psychological tests. They suggest this discrepancy is a consequence of denial on the part of sufferers, resulting in normative responses to standard screening tools, whilst focal questionnaires reveal the extent of their difficulties.

The study is important, since it focuses on the area of social difficulty, a matter of specific concern to this group. However, the study also appears to examine many elements which relate not to current distress, but to past experiences and perceptions of the attitudes of others. These are not necessarily indicative of current distress. Thus, it is not necessarily the case that responses to this questionnaire are either different from the findings of standard tests, or more revealing about current psychological adjustment. It is quite possible that the responses are different because they are measuring different things, rather than because of denial or other concealment by the respondent. Similarly, the authors were comparing global abnormality on the HAD and GHQ with single-item responses to their questionnaire. This seems an inadequate method of comparison between the two methods of assessment. Thus, there is no reason to conclude that standardised tests are failing to detect psychological disturbance when it is present. Moreover, Newell (2000) demonstrated that GHQ and HAD did indeed reveal psychological disturbance to be present in facially disfigured people, to a greater extent than in the general population.

Severity and location of disfigurement as predictors of psychosocial disturbance

It may be, as Piff suggested (Holmes 1986), that professionals underestimate the level of disturbance experienced by people with facial disfigurements. The lack of concordance between level of injury and level of psychological disturbance is often mentioned in the literature, and indeed is cited by Pruzinsky (1992) as one of the most consistent findings in the field of body image study. Moreover, preoccupation by patients with what is regarded by health professionals as minimal disfigurement is often taken as a sign of psychopathology. Nevertheless, criteria for determining an acceptable level of disfigurement do not exist, the number of studies examining extent and site of disfigurement as variables possibly affecting psychosocial adjustment is small, and the conclusions regarding the impact of level and site of disfigurement on adjustment are mixed.

Andreason and Norris's (1972) examination of adjustment in burns provides a detailed tabular account of the areas of injury suffered by the subjects. This is particularly important in judging the authors' assertion that their results offer some support for Macgregor *et al.*'s (1953) suggestion that patients with less deformity may be more disturbed. As has been noted earlier, numbers in the Andreason and Norris (1972) study were small, and so any suggestion that general trends about behaviour and experience might be drawn from it should be modest. Furthermore, although the authors *suggest* that some of their results support Macgregor *et al.* (1953), this is not apparent when the data are scrutinised. Examination of the tabular results shows that of those judged to have emotional problems, only one had an examiner-rated level of disfigurement of less than 3 on a 1 to 4 scale, with 4 representing maximum disfigurement level, and this individual *self*-rated at 3. Likewise, visual inspection of the relationship between ratings of disfigurement level and poor adjustment indicates that these appear to be *positively* rather than negatively related. Thus, inspection of Andreason and Norris's (1972) data does not support their conclusion that these data add weight to Macgregor *et al.*'s (1953) contention that lower levels of disfigurement are associated with higher levels of disturbance. Indeed, the data appear to refute it – those with high levels of difficulty have amongst the highest ratings of disfigurement.

In an important study of psychosocial adjustment amongst burns survivors, Browne *et al.* (1985) examined previous studies in the area and found only three which were not weakened by design difficulties, small sample size, or biases in approach to sampling or measurement. Their own study attempted to assess levels and predictors of psychosocial adjustment in burns victims. They gave 340 randomly selected adult burn survivors and the parents of 145 child burn survivors with either major or minor burns a battery of validated questionnaire measures, in order to determine whether adjustment was affected by severity of and time since the injury, coping methods and social resources. In adults, they found that poor adjustment was associated with avoidance coping, little use of logical analysis or problem-solving, high information-seeking, affective distance from life problems, recency of burn, fewer recreations, and less perceived family, friend and peer support. Extent of the burn made no difference to adjustment. In the child sample, there was again no association between size of burn and adjustment, but mothers of less adjusted children demonstrated greater avoidance coping, affective distance, fewer recreations and less moral or religious emphasis within the family. The presence of avoidance and poor problem-solving were the most consistent explanatory factors with regard to poor psychosocial adjustment. It is tempting, therefore, to suggest that this study offers support for a behavioural approach to the amelioration of psychological difficulties following burn disfigurement, given the emphasis within behaviour therapy upon problem-solving and confrontation.

Love *et al.* (1987), in an investigation of whether individuals burned in childhood were less well adjusted than others as adults, did attempt to distinguish between levels of disfigurement amongst their 42 burns survivor subjects, to whom they administered the Billings and Moos Coping Scale and the Psychosocial Adjustment to Illness Scale (PAIS). All had scores within the normal range, indicating that all were well adjusted, and there were no differences according to severity of the burn. However, dividing the group at the median PAIS score revealed a difference in interviewer ratings of their level of disfigurement. The less disfigured were better adjusted ($X^2 = 10.21$, $P = 0.01$). The distinction is, however, somewhat dubious, since the whole group was well adjusted!

In a follow-up of burned patients, Blumenfield and Reddish (1987) identified 16 patients who were unable to resume their jobs or social activities after several months and also had symptoms of psychological disturbance, from a group of sixty-eight patients with mild/moderate burn injuries. Using a database of 250 questionnaire items, the authors compared these 'small burn, big problem (SBBP)' patients with others who did not have difficulties. They reported no differences in age, sex, race, length of stay, circumstances of injury, extent of burn or amount of disfigurement between the groups. There were, however, significant differences on measures of regression, displacement and seeing injury as a narcissistic threat. The mechanism of displacement was regarded by the authors as important because they state it is a major component of phobic behaviour. Many of the SBBP patients were identified as phobic.

Unfortunately, the study is weakened by lack of description of the development of the scale. The 250 items were simply noted as being related to the study variables in previous literature, and no account of the instrument's validity or reliability is given. The patients' difficulties were elicited via interview, but no discussion of possible bias is given. The manner of operationalising and identifying regression, narcissism and displacement from interview is not described. A considerable number of comparisons appear possible, and we do not know how many were made prior to reporting, and therefore if those actually reported were likely to be artefacts of the number of comparisons made, and significance levels are given without a note of the tests employed. The data themselves are inadequately reported. In consequence, no firm conclusions regarding any relationship between extent of burn and psychological disturbance can be made.

The role of the face in determining psychosocial difficulty after burns is supported in Williams and Griffiths's (1991) examination of adjustment in 23 representative burns patients from a series of 55. They administered the Hospital Anxiety and Depression Scale (HADS), Impact of Event Scale (IES) and a series of questions related to the burn itself to respondents in an attempt to ascertain both the extent and nature of psychosocial difficulties and the possibility of being able to predict them from patient variables. They found three HADS depression and eight HADS anxiety cases and four IES avoidance and three IES intrusion cases 1 year after discharge, and found that the best predictor of difficulty was visibility of the area. Both hands and face were included on the visibility scale, but the authors note that the greatest number of patients expressing difficulties came from the 'face only' group, and conclude that it is likely that facial involvement is the best predictor of psychosocial difficulty.

Whilst the numbers in this study are small to justify such an assertion, taken along with the similar finding by Roca *et al.* (1992) it may be argued that there is support for the belief that facial involvement is a major cause of post-burn psychosocial disturbance. It is likewise interesting to speculate that much of the disturbance found in studies which do not differentiate according to site of the burn may also be caused by facial disfigurement, and particularly unfortunate that these studies have not allowed a more definitive examination of the role played by different parts of the body in determining psychosocial adjustment.

However, such a speculation is weakened by the findings of Blakeney *et al.*'s (1988) study of adjustment in 38 burns patients. Although the numbers were again small, these workers found no differences between individuals with ($n = 20$) and without ($n = 18$) facial burns, when examined at least 2 years after the burn according to a battery of validated instruments. Nor did severity of the burn predict greater psychological disturbance. However, the use of the Suicide Probability Scale to determine adjustment may be both imprecise and less than comprehensive.

Nevertheless, further support for the notion that locus or severity of burn do not predict adjustment is provided in a study by Orr *et al.* (1989), who found no effect of locus of burn injury on the body image and self-esteem of 121 burn-injured adolescents and young adults. They noted that the evidence regarding relationships between locus of burn injury and self-esteem was equivocal, although depression after illness had been found to be greater when the illness or disfigurement was visible, and related to total body surface area affected in burns (Chang and Hertzog 1976). Nevertheless, their own study, which had expected lower self-esteem, less positive body image and greater depression amongst those burned on socially sensitive (i.e. visible) areas, found no such relationships. Nor were these variables associated with time elapsed since the burn or total body surface area burned. The relationship between burns and psychosocial adjustment is clearly more complex than the influence of a single factor such as site of the burn.

An earlier study by White (1982) examined the effects of area of burn and gender on psychological disturbance, using both a clinical assessment and an adaptation of the GHQ to assess psychological change between the accident and 1 year follow-up in 142 burn victims and 136 age- and sex-matched victims of non-burn accidents. Burns patients had a non-significant trend towards greater psychological disturbance than non-burns patients, but there was no difference according to area of burn, with the single exception that males with leg burns had fewer difficulties than other groups. However, severity of injury was predictive of disturbance.

If site of burn does not always predict later adjustment, the salience of the face as a determinant of such adjustment (and the possible speculation that it plays a role in descriptions of such adjustment in elements of the burns literature which do not differentiate according to site) is suggested strongly by Hughes *et al.*'s (1983) study of dermatology patients. Administration of GHQ thirty to 196 outpatients and forty inpatients revealed that 30% of the outpatients and 60% of the inpatients had high scores, with a higher level than the general population and general hospital inpatients respectively. Most importantly to the discussion of the relevance of site to psychological disturbance, 70% of patients with hand and face involvement ($n = 47$) showed high scores. Furthermore, disfigurement and stigma, along with inconvenience, were the most frequently cited causes of the psychiatric symptoms reported by high scorers, whilst some 34% of high scorers reported avoiding people.

The importance of the face in determining psychological reactions to illness is underlined by other dermatological studies. Shuster *et al.* (1978) examined the role of skin complaints in self-image, asking acne, eczema and psoriasis sufferers and normal controls to rate schematic faces previously scored by independent judges on such characteristics as happiness, intelligence and good looks. Subjects rated the pictures on such dimensions as 'like me', 'like someone I like', or 'me in 10 years' time'. Their perceptions of the pictures might thus be taken as indices of their self-image. Whilst controls demonstrated correlations between judges' ratings of characteristics such as good-looking and likeable and ratings of 'like me' and 'desirable', in the acne patients there was a significant decrease in correlations with positive attributes of the pictures as acne severity increased, with similarly increasing correlations with attributes of 'someone I dislike', more markedly affecting females. Eczema and psoriasis sufferers were less severely affected, a difference the authors attribute to the possibility of differing sites of the complaints, although no note of site is recorded.

That psychological difficulties are related to visibility to others is suggested by Porter *et al.*'s (1986) comparison of vitiligo patients with controls and psoriasis sufferers. All subjects rated lower than controls on a validated measure of self-esteem, but psoriasis sufferers reported significantly more discrimination against them than vitiligo sufferers, including being stared at and job discrimination. They were also more likely to report embarrassment, and scored lower on a measure of adjustment to the disorder. Psoriasis sufferers were less likely to use make-up as camouflage, presumably because their complaint involves changes in skin texture and skin lesions, rather than simple pigmentary change. Thus visibility was increased in the psoriasis group.

Modest further support for the role of the face in determining psychosocial adjustment is found in a study of recovery after treatment of cystic acne. Rubinow *et al.* (1987) suggested that clinical experience indicates that acne sufferers report self-consciousness and fear of social rejection and are socially isolated and limited in their activities owing to embarrassment and mental or physical discomfort. They examined fifty-five sufferers using a range of questionnaires and found that whilst pain from the lesions was a major difficulty for 55% of respondents, some 91% reported embarrassment, whilst 40% noted self-consciousness, 29% social isolation and 20% anxiety with the opposite sex. A subject group of sixty-six patients also scored higher than normals on the Hopkins Symptom Checklist, but lower than psychiatric patients. Whilst none of these scores differed between those with facial lesions and the rest of the group, those with facial lesions did show greater improvement in depression following treatment. However, this effect is perhaps confounded by the fact that patients with facial lesions also showed greater dermatological improvement.

There are difficulties in examining the psychosocial difficulties of head and neck cancer patients in relation to disfigurement, because many other factors contribute to their difficulties (e.g. difficulties with speaking and eating, fear of a life-threatening complaint). However, a study by Cassileth *et al.* (1983) of the impact of differing levels of disfigurement on melanoma patients' perceptions of the cosmetic impact of their operations focused specifically on disfigurement. They administered questionnaires to 181 patients, obtaining their opinions of the size and cosmetic impact of wide lesion excision scars. As well as completing a ten-item report of the impact of the scar, subjects drew the size of their scar on a figure outline in a method similar to that of Rumsey (1983). Clinic nurses assessed the degree of indentation associated with graft closures. The major findings were that although length of scar did not distinguish between high and low impact individuals, the highest impact group were distinguished from lowest impact by greater degree of indentation, type of closure (graft) and lack of correspondence between expected and actual scar size (where this was larger). Patients' drawings corresponded well with actual size of scars (a ratio of 1.01 where 1.0 would be perfect), indicating that disfigured individuals have an accurate perception of their bodily appearance. Women were significantly more distressed than men even though their scars were smaller.

There are, however, some difficulties with the study, since the statistical tests used are not described adequately. Moreover, although the authors describe the correlations noted as 'significant', they do not give correlation coefficients, and so we cannot tell how large the correlations were. Finally, there were difficulties with some of the scales used. The rating of surgical indentation used a three-point ordinal scale (none, moderate, severe), yet measures of central tendency and spread based on an interval level of measurement (mean and standard deviation) are used, leading one to suspect that the inferential tests employed might have been parametric tests, which would likewise have been inappropriate. The expectation of scar scale is unlikely to be valid, since it contained only the following possible responses: 'not larger', 'a little larger', 'somewhat larger' and 'a lot larger'. Respondents thus had no opportunity to state that they expected a smaller scar than that which in fact resulted from the operation, with the resultant possibility of skewing in favour of expectation of larger scars. Finally, there was no investigation of any difference made by site of the scar, although this may impact upon ratings of level of disfigurement (Dropkin et al. 1983). Nevertheless, the possibility that expectation might affect perception of impact has possible implications for preparation for surgery, and merits further investigation.

If the ratings were suspect in the above study, the investigation by Baker (1992) represents a careful attempt to distinguish between levels of facial disfigurement, in examining the effect of differences in such levels on rehabilitation of head and neck cancer patients. Fifty-one patients completed a self-report questionnaire regarding twelve activities of daily living. Baker rated patients' level of disfigurement by comparing their operation site with Dropkin et al.'s (1983) position/severity scale. However, the study found no correlation between either a total score of rehabilitation based on activities of daily living or its physical or psychological dimensions and level of facial disfigurement. There was a correlation between the eating item of the questionnaire and disfigurement. The absence of other correlations with disfigurement might also be explained by the general low to moderate levels of disfigurement (mean of 3.9 from a 0–11 scale), which might have decreased the likelihood of finding differences. This study represents one of few studies which focused specifically on facial disfigurement *and* used a sufficiently robust method to allow us to have confidence in accuracy of its failure to find a relationship between severity of disfigurement and subsequent rehabilitation, including measures of psychological functioning.

A further study of head and neck patients, by Gamba et al. (1992), also focused specifically on disfigurement. The authors compared groups of patients with minor versus extensive disfigurements. Although the method of classification was dubious, being based on 'evident perception of facial deformity' by the clinician, the authors also took account of type and site of surgery, using Dropkin *et al.*'s (1983) approach to classification, and all patients had tumours of greater than 3 cm removed. Sixty-six patients were interviewed at between 6 months and 8 years post surgery. Those with extensive disfigurement reported greater change to self-image, worse relationships with partner, reduced sexuality, and increased social isolation, whilst 18% of respondents felt the disadvantages of treatment outweighed the advantages. Self-image was cited as the most important change by more respondents with extensive than with minor disfigurement, and those with extensive disfigurement were more likely to avoid touching the operation area, avoid looking in mirrors and to no longer feel attractive. Of those reporting major disadvantages following treatment, 79% were accounted for by patients who felt differently about their body image.

Attempts to establish the existence or otherwise of a relationship between severity of change to bodily appearance and psychological disturbance are important to our understanding of the experiences of disfigured people and the targeting of those potentially most at risk from psychosocial difficulties. An important element of this may be the education of the medical and nursing professions with regard to both these experiences and potential risk factors. Assertions of a negative relationship between level of disfigurement and level of psychosocial disturbance should currently be strongly resisted, particularly given the tendency to ascribe psychopathology to individuals describing psychosocial disturbance or requesting medical and surgical interventions to ameliorate facial abnormalities. This assertion is frequently made and is potentially damaging to disfigured people. The literature simply does not support it once it is subjected to close scrutiny. Macgregor *et al.*'s (1953) assertion of this negative relationship comes very early in her extensive exploration of this area, and is based on clinical impression alone, whilst the studies which purport to support it are flawed with regard to both method (Blumenfeld and Reddish 1987; Blakeney *et al.* 1988) and interpretation (Andreason and Norris 1972). There is, therefore, likewise no support for the proposition suggested by Reich (1969) that this supposed greater disturbance in less disfigured individuals results from the unpredictability of people's reactions to them. It appears that the most conservative assessment of the literature is that no relationship has been proved. However, several studies directly suggest that greater disfigurement might be associated with *worse* adjustment (Chang and Hertzog 1976; White 1982; Cassileth *et al.* 1983; Gamba *et al.* 1992).

Moreover, close examination of the Andreason and Norris data likewise supports this position. With regard to site of disfigurement, there seems reasonable support for the notions that visibility and, in particular, facial involvement are associated with worse adjustment. It might be speculated that these studies in fact offer indirect support for the notion of a relationship between high disfigurement and high levels of disturbance, if we regard visibility of the change in appearance as an index of level of disfigurement.

Other predictors of psychosocial difficulties following disfigurement

Examination of the effect of level of severity and site of the disfigurement represents one tactic in attempting to predict who will develop psychosocial difficulties following disfigurement. Many of the studies in this area investigate numerous different variables, and so there is some overlap between this and the previous section. In general, however, the current section examines the possible effect of gender, personality variables and social support amongst disfigured people upon their psychosocial well-being. Personal variables of this kind are of importance in informing fear–avoidance models of pain and of body image disturbance (Lethem *et al.* 1983; Newell 1991, 1999; Slade 1994, and see Chapter 3).

Gender is perhaps the most extensively investigated of these variables, and it has been suggested that females suffer greater psychosocial disturbance, possibly as a result of the greater emphasis placed by society on female appearance (Andreason and Norris 1972). Whilst Andreason and Norris argued that women in their own study did indeed show greater disturbance, this assertion was based on extremely small numbers (four women versus two men showing 'complications'). The study by Orr *et al.* (1989) described earlier offers some support for their contention. Females in the Orr *et al.* study had more negative body image, depression and lower self-esteem than males. By contrast, the White (1982) study did not find differences between men and women.

A major study by Brown *et al.* (1988) also focused on gender and psychosocial difficulties. In their study of 260 burned individuals (209 males and fifty-one females), functional disability, disfigurement, coping responses and social resources were examined for their effect on adjustment. They used validated measures of coping and adjustment and rated disfigurement on a scale which ran from no visible scarring through several gradations of altered skin texture to missing body parts or facial disfigurement. Both males and females were generally found to be adjusted, whilst high levels of adjustment were correlated with less functional disability in males and greater problem-solving in women. Females used more cognitive coping and information-seeking than males. Psychological adjustment to illness was the same across genders, with the exception of a vocational disruption subscale, which showed more disruption in females. Multiple regression investigated which combinations of variables best explained psychological adjustment. A combination of low functional disability, more recreational activities, greater friend support, less avoidance coping, and more problem-solving accounted together for 55% of variance. In men less functional disability was the most important predictor of adjustment, whilst in women the most important factor was problem-solving.

It may be concluded from this study that some variables associated with better psychosocial adjustment are different between the sexes, although the overall effect of disfigurement on adjustment is not different across the genders. This finding, the authors note, does not confirm Andreason and Norris's (1972) contention regarding gender and disfigurement. The findings of this study also suggest that variables associated with tactics often employed in cognitive-behaviour therapy (non-avoidance, problem-solving, recreational activity) are likewise implicated in better adjustment.

A physical variable which might be expected to distinguish between more and less psychological disturbance amongst disfigured people is level of attractiveness. Starr (1980) examined the effect of facial attractiveness on the behaviour of forty-nine patients with cleft lips, cleft palates and cleft lips and palates. Subjects were given structured measures of behaviour and of self-esteem, and their scores compared according to attractiveness. There were no differences between matched scarred and non-scarred subjects, nor any between the attractive and unattractive groups. However, no subject gained a rating of over 15/20 on the rating scale used by the investigators, indicating that none of the subjects was highly attractive. This might lead us to conclude that the lack of significant differences between attractive and unattractive individuals was an artefact of the subjects occupying less than the total range of possible different attractiveness levels. Splitting the group into two on the basis of high and low attractiveness ratings which were quite close to each other may have lessened the sensitivity of the study's ability to detect differences between the groups.

The role of demographic factors in mediating adjustment is supported by results of the White (1982) study mentioned earlier, which found greater difficulty amongst those with pre-existing anxiety, depression or personality disorder, in the age range 36–45 and living alone or with three children. A further study by Tucker (1987) examined several possible predictive factors in determining psychosocial difficulties in burns survivors, and suggested the role of personality variables such as neuroticism, trait anxiety and hypochondriasis, as well as individual variations such as the presence of pre-morbid psychiatric disorder, post-traumatic stress disorder (PTSD), compensation claims and severity of the burn. From this study of thirty-one patients, Tucker notes that depression and anxiety are moderately elevated in pre-discharge patients but drop to normal or low levels with the passage of time, whilst there is a significant incidence of PTSD. However, neither PTSD nor severity of burn were predictors of psychosocial difficulty (although numbers were very small for such comparisons), whilst the personality variables which predicted difficulty yielded moderate correlations at best.

A later investigation of the role of PTSD (Roca et al. 1992) in post-burn adjustment obtained a slightly larger sample ($n = 41$) and examined them at discharge and 4 month follow-up. PTSD was found in 7% of patients at discharge and 22% at follow-up, but was not strongly associated with poor psychosocial adjustment. This is one of comparatively few studies to identify area and type of burn specifically. Whilst neither of these variables was associated with level of PTSD symptoms, facial involvement was correlated with low scores on the social (0.68) and sexual adaptation (0.65) domains of the survey, lending further support to the notion, suggested in the previous section, that visibility is associated with greater difficulty.

Moore et al. (1993) suggested that personality traits might predict adjustment following changes to people's lives caused by burns. To test this, they gave thirty-two patients a validated measure of personality and divided them into well adjusted and poorly adjusted according to the Suicide Probability Scale (SPS). They noted that patients regarded as well adjusted on this basis had significantly higher scores on the H scale (which measures a tendency towards boldness and impulsivity) and on a higher order factor of 'extroversion'. However, a measure of emotional lability did not significantly differentiate between the groups, resulting in only a non-significant trend towards such a differentiation. The authors conclude that specific character traits 'seem to be' related to adjustment after burns, although they are careful not to attribute any causality, owing to the regression paradigm used to examine the relationships. However, their study comprised small numbers.

The role of social support as a determinant of better adjustment is suggested by a survey by Davidson *et al.* (1981) of 314 burns-injured people treated over the course of 20 years. Respondents were interviewed using a 519-item schedule which ranged from socio-economic variables to satisfaction with treatment, and also measured life satisfaction, self-esteem, participation in social and recreational activities and social support. Severity of injury was also rated, but site of the injury was not reported.

Social support was found to be related to life satisfaction ($r = 0.37$), self-esteem ($r = 0.40$) and social and recreational participation ($r = 0.14$). The authors conclude that identification of the patient's social network is important in facilitating rehabilitation. It is interesting to note, however, that the correlation between support and social and recreational activity, though significant, was extremely modest.

Addressing the psychosocial difficulties of facially disfigured people

The descriptions of social interaction by and with disfigured people given earlier in this and previous chapters, and the potentially negative consequences of such interactions, indicate that intervention to alter the quality of such interactions is potentially an important contribution to the lives of disfigured people. However, the systematic investigation of treatment of psychosocial consequences of disfigurement is in its infancy. Facial disfigurement has been the subject of little research, and psychological treatment is even less thoroughly investigated, despite the fact that the difficulties of facially disfigured people have been described, at least in anecdotal form, in the literature since at least the early works of Macgregor in the 1950s.

In view of this it is surprising to find that more recent accounts of both the extent of treatment provision and the interventions themselves remain extremely rare. It must be presumed that they reflect an actual treatment provision which is equally fragmented and inadequate. Two surveys from the 1980s reported a lack of focus upon emotional difficulties. Wallace (1988), in a study of forty-threeUnited Kingdom burns units, found that, of the twenty-eight replies received, only two units provided specialist counselling, whilst only seven had some form of lay support. This lack of emphasis on emotional support was also seen in a US study (Kaplan 1985), which found that only 70% of burns units gave *any* information about emotional aspects of burn injuries. It will be remembered from earlier in this chapter that Wallace (1988) also found that almost all the burns patients in her survey of their psychosocial needs reported a desire for some form of emotional intervention or support, whilst less than 25% reported *any* useful contact with any professional with regard to their burns. Many of her findings regarding identified psychological intervention needs were confirmed by Williams and Griffiths (1991). Further, larger surveys of the psychosocial needs of disfigured people and provision to meet these needs would now be timely, particularly since informal contacts with specialist nurses indicate that the position has improved somewhat since the time of these studies.

Studies of the role of psychiatrists and psychologists focus chiefly on assessment of suitability for surgery (Jacobson *et al.* 1961), general liaison roles within plastic surgery units (Goin and Goin 1981) and descriptions of psychological difficulties such as those described in this chapter. Accounts of treatment are almost exclusively restricted to single case studies or collections of such studies (Jacobson *et al.* 1961; Bernstein 1976, 1982; Cohen *et al.* 1991; Shakin Kunkel *et al.* 1995), or to general descriptions of therapeutic approaches (Bronheim *et al.* 1991). These studies do not always differentiate between pre-existing psychological difficulties and the consequences of disfigurement, nor between the consequences of the disfiguring aspects of impairments and functional aspects such as difficulty with speech and eating following oral surgery. Some include patients with active or terminal malignant disease, and likewise focus on a broad range of issues. They are thus not studies of therapy for disfigurement, and are not discussed here.

As noted in Chapter 4, Lefebvre and Arndt (1988) outlined psychological protective factors in disfigurement. They also suggested a number of tactics which might be employed to increase life skills in adolescents with facial disfigurements, based on 15 years of liaison psychiatry in this area. These included: helping strangers handle shock and fear, handling teasing and name-calling, making new friends, talking to members of the opposite sex, handling job interviews. Unfortunately, although their review is extensively referenced, none of these citations refers to therapeutic intervention. In consequence, their account of these interventions remains at an anecdotal level, and no conclusion can be drawn about the effectiveness or otherwise of the treatment suggestions they make, which are further weakened by inadequate description of the interventions undertaken.

One study specifically addresses the social skills of disfigured individuals (Feigenbaum 1981), in the context of a 'social training' programme which also included elements of anxiety reduction, following Meichenbaum's (1977) stress inoculation approach to cognitive-behaviour therapy. Although the groups were not analysed using a statistical model which would allow direct comparison of differences in the changes between the two groups over time, the results demonstrated significant differences both between pre- and post-training scores for the experimental group, and between the experimental and control groups post treatment across a variety of measures of anxiety. The analysis would have been strengthened by the inclusion of data from the initial time point for the control group, and by the examination of any possible effects of differences between experimental and control groups pre-treatment. Despite this methodological weakness, the range and number of significant results which favour the intervention allow us to have reasonable confidence in its effectiveness.

The lack of systematic examination of psychosocial interventions with people with facial disfigurements, and the absence, with the exception of the Feigenbaum (1981) study, of attempts specifically to address issues of social isolation, mean that the work of Rumsey, Partridge and their various collaborators is particularly welcome. Partridge is a burns survivor who has developed an approach to treatment based on a group approach which involves social skills training of the kind advocated by Rumsey (1983) but also such diverse elements as role modelling, imitation, instruction, brainstorming, role plays, creative problem-solving and feedback (Partridge 1993). His approach is clearly focused on the interpersonal consequences of disfigurement, which are outlined in the 'scared' model of reactions (see Table 6.1). Workshops address elements of this 'scared' responding.

The workshops are now part of a continuing programme of therapeutic evaluation which builds on Rumsey's research work (Rumsey 1983; Rumsey et al. 1986a) and Partridge's personal experiences (Partridge 1990) and work with social skills training. In a review of this group's work to date, Partridge et al. (1994) note that the 'Changing Faces' project had developed a series of workshops for disfigured people which, during the first two years of the project, some 88% of attenders found useful, whilst 77% reported using the skills and information they had gained on the course in real life situations.

In a further account of the work of the project (Robinson et al. 1996), a consecutive series of 112 attenders at 'Changing Faces' workshops were examined using the HADS and the Social Avoidance and Distress Scale (SADS) as well as open-ended questions regarding quality of life. Respondents reported difficulties in social situations, particularly with regard to meeting new people and being with strangers. Of the original group, 64 completed both a 6 week and a 6 month follow-up. Six weeks after the workshops, HADS anxiety had fallen significantly, and was no

Table 6.1 The 'scared' syndrome

You		They	
feel	*behave*	*feel*	*behave*
self-conscious	submissive	sympathy	staring
conspicuous	clumsy	caution	curiosity
angry	apathy	anguished	awkwardness
resentful	regressive	reluctant	rudeness
empty	excluded	embarrassed	evasiveness
different	defenceless	dread	distance

Source: Partridge (1993).

longer different from normative samples. Similarly, high levels of SADS social avoidance and distress had significantly reduced after treatment, and attenders felt significantly more confident in the presence of strangers and when meeting new people. Improvements were maintained or increased at 6 month follow-up. Age of participants and duration of disfigurement were unrelated to extent of psychological difficulties both before and after treatment. The study lacks a control group, but the comparison with normative data on the HADS increases confidence that participant improvements represent a genuine effect, although the possibility that this improvement is an artefact of attention or time cannot definitively be refuted.

The authors conclude that social skills training workshops offer a 'promising' intervention. Whilst this is certainly an appropriately conservative assertion, given that the study represents an uncontrolled design, it should be considered within the context both of the levels of improvement reported and of the current lack of any other systematic studies. Taking this into account, social skills training represents the most important step to date towards addressing the psychological difficulties of disfigured people. Whilst caution should be urged, in the light for example of Bernstein's (1976) remarks regarding the possible arrogance of assuming that such social manipulations could materially change the psychological well-being of disfigured people, two factors should give increased cause for optimism. First, despite its simplicity as an intervention, social skills training has a considerable record of clinical effectiveness across a broad variety of difficulties. Second, the workshops organised by Partridge's group appear to offer a flexible, eclectic approach to social skills training which goes beyond the simple training of interaction skills via role play, to include brainstorming and creative problem-solving. Whilst there is little specific reference to anxiety management, the inference is clear that anxiety reduction is an aim of the workshops, whose key elements appear to be rooted firmly within the cognitive-behavioural tradition.

There is some suggestion that recognition of the value of such a behaviourally oriented approach has filtered into the therapeutic awareness of health professionals. Griffiths (1990), writing before publication of the 'Changing Faces' project's work, suggested a series of tactics a nurse might use in helping disfigured people. These included:

- not giving in to avoidance
- using controlled breathing to control fear and anxiety
- using positive self-talk
- concentrating on relevant information to distract from upsetting thoughts
- avoiding misinterpreting the discomfort of others as rejection
- finding a way to acknowledge the disfigurement
- congratulating success.

These suggestions are once again clearly rooted in cognitive-behavioural interventions, but this is not specifically acknowledged in Griffiths's (1990) article. Nor are any of the suggestions referenced. There is no sign from the nursing or medical literature that either these suggestions or any other cognitive-behavioural interventions have been adopted.

Treatment provision for the psychosocial consequences of disfigurement has been subjected only to the most minimal investigation, but appears rudimentary. There is little description of the role of psychiatrists, psychologists or specialist nurses in the provision of care to disfigured people. Considerable numbers of disfigured people appear not to have the benefit of contact with services designed to address their psychosocial needs. Description of treatment interventions to date has been sketchy. The only systematic programme of work is that of the Rumsey/Partridge group in the field of social skills training. Although work in social skills training is hampered by the lack of adequately controlled trials, this work still shows considerable promise, with apparent benefit to disfigured people. The treatment programmes appear to contain several elements of a cognitive-behavioural approach. This approach to treatment is also implicitly suggested in Griffiths's (1990) paper. However, empirical investigation of her suggestions is lacking.

In the chapter which follows a number of empirical tests of the fear–avoidance model of psychological difficulty following disfigurement are presented. As part of this series of tests, a controlled study of a cognitive-behavioural self-help intervention (Newell 2000) is described.

Exercise

Little description of initiatives to offer psychological support to people who have experienced a change in body image is available in the published literature. Find out what initiatives are available in your area, both in hospitals and in primary care settings. Find out what efforts have been made to publicise them and to share the skills involved.

Key further reading

Andreason, N. and Norris, A. (1972) Long-term adjustment and adaptation mechanisms in severely burned adults. *Journal of Nervous and Mental Disease* 154(5), 352–62.

Andreason, N., Norris, A. and Hartford, L. (1971) Incidence of long-term psychiatric complication in severely burned adults. *Annals of Surgery* 174, 785–93.

Flawed early accounts of the psychological consequences of burns and disfigurement. It is important that these early studies are read critically, since their (often erroneous) conclusions have been followed by some later authors.

Partridge, J., Coutinho, W., Robinson, E. and Rumsey, N. (1994) Changing Faces: two years on. *Nursing Standard* 18 May, 8(34), 54–8.

Robinson, E., Rumsey, N. and Partridge, J. (1996) An evaluation of the impact of social interaction skills training for facially disfigured people. *British Journal of Plastic Surgery* 49, 281–9.

Two reports of the work of the 'Changing Faces' group.

Part 3

Using the cognitive-behavioural approach to disturbed body image

Chapter 7

Support for a cognitive-behavioural approach

In Part 1, the problem of body image disturbance was examined, several possible models were identified, and their strengths and weaknesses outlined. A cognitive-behavioural model of body image and its disturbance was presented, with a particular emphasis on fear and avoidance as mediating factors in determining the extent of adaptation following a threat to body image such as disfigurement. It was noted that previous models of disturbed body image have undergone little empirical testing. In Part 2, a context for the development and potential importance of such models was provided, through an examination of some of the research literature relevant to disfigurement, its psychological consequences and their treatment. In this chapter, we will now examine the likely extent of support for the fear–avoidance model advanced in Chapter 3. This will include indirect support (from studies not directly related to the model, but whose results suggest that it might be useful) and direct support (from a series of studies (Newell 1998, 1999, 2000; Newell and Clarke 2000; Newell and Marks 2000) intended specifically to test the assumptions made by a fear–avoidance model of psychological difficulty following disfigurement).

Indirect support for the cognitive-behavioural approach to treatment of disturbed body image and disfigurement

Prior to the Newell series, there were no published studies of the treatment of psychological sequelae of disfigurement from a specifically cognitive-behavioural viewpoint, with the exception of Robinson *et al.*'s (1996) study and the studies of Feigenbaum (1981), both of which focus on social skills training as the main treatment element. These offer limited support for the cognitive-behavioural approach, to the extent that we might be able to infer from their success that fear and avoidance might be the variables being affected during the treatment of participants in these studies. This, however, is indeed limited, since there is neither any specific reference to the use of exposure therapies in addressing social or other behavioural avoidances in disfigured individuals, nor mention of the role that such therapies might play in illuminating the processes which mediate the psychosocial difficulties of disfigured people.

There are, however, studies of cognitive-behavioural interventions in areas of relevance to disfigurement, if we assume the occurrence of social avoidance and body image dissatisfaction in disfigurement. The main treatment studies which bear upon these difficulties are in the area of social phobia, eating disorders and, most recently, body dysmorphic disorder. Social phobia was examined in Chapter 3, but it is worth noting again that this client problem is relevant to treatment of disfigured individuals because of the social difficulties they experience, provided it is possible to demonstrate that these difficulties are phobic in nature, and therefore amenable to cognitive-behavioural intervention.

A great deal of work in the area of body image has come from studies of *disturbance* of body image in general, and from studies of eating disorders in particular. Much of the treatment of such disturbance has likewise been conducted in the area of eating disorders, an area in which cognitive-behavioural interventions are now pre-eminent, in terms both of amount of study devoted to them, and of the success of their approaches.

Treatment of eating disorders, in particular anorexia nervosa and bulimia, by behavioural means has a long history (Fairburn and Cooper 1989). The relevance of such treatments to disfigured people lies in the negative appraisal of their body by sufferers of anorexia and bulimia, and in their behavioural avoidances. Negative body appraisal and body image distortion by people with eating disorders were noted in Chapter 2. The behavioural avoidances of anorexia in particular are a distinctive feature, and the complaint has variously been described as a weight phobia (Crisp 1967) and a fear of fatness (Russell 1970), as well as possessing obsessional features (Fairburn and Cooper 1989). The chief avoidances are of eating and weight gain, whilst there are often such other avoidances as specific foods, eating in front of others, or wearing revealing clothes. All these avoidances are said to be fuelled by the inappropriate perception of ideal body size and negative appraisal of the sufferer's own body. Other clinical features such as vomiting, abuse of purgative agents, dieting and extreme exercise are likewise considered to be secondary to these overvalued ideas regarding appropriate shape and weight. However, clinicians in the field both acknowledge the importance of other difficulties less obviously related to body image (e.g. disordered family functioning, fear of loss of control), and address these issues during treatment. Thus, extrapolations from treatment of people with eating disorders to those with disfigurement should be made with caution, and this literature will not be examined here. The cognitive-behaviour therapy (CBT) approach is well summarised by Fairburn and Cooper (1989) and involves a variety of elements such as retraining eating habits, the use of stimulus control techniques, cognitive restructuring and self-monitoring, many of which involve the client in exposure to feared situations such as weight gain, shape change and eating. Most recently, the cognitive-behavioural approach has been recognised nationally as the psychological treatment with the greatest chance of success in bulimia (Department of Health 1999).

The success of CBT in addressing bulimia and other eating disorders is relevant to the study of psychosocial difficulty following disfigurement because of the presence within these disorders of both disturbance of body image and the behavioural avoidances which are said to be consequences of this disturbance. A pattern of disturbed body image and behavioural avoidance has also been found in body dysmorphic disorder (BDD), the psychological disorder which perhaps has most in common with psychological difficulty following disfigurement or other change to bodily appearance or function. This complaint, referred to as dysmorphophobia in earlier studies but described as BDD throughout this review, is an irrational fear that a bodily attribute is offensive to others. Since the complaint usually centres around a single attribute, such as a facial feature, the growing success of CBT in treatment is of particular potential importance with reference to psychosocial difficulties following disfigurement.

Although some commentators have denied that BDD is truly phobic, since the body attribute is not itself feared, Hay (1970) rightly comments that the phobic element is present, but in the patient's fear of offending others aesthetically. It is interesting, in this connection, to recall the fear of negative appraisal by others present in social phobia. It likewise seems possible that this fear is also present in disfigured people, given the amount of time they are reputed to spend checking the possible reactions of others (Macgregor et al. 1953). It may be possible that the fear of offending others in body dysmorphic disorder might be prepared for in Seligman's (1971) sense of having species survival value in the same way that was suggested of socially phobic fears in Chapter 3. The existence of the attractiveness stereotype described in Chapter 4 and the great importance attached to physical, and particularly facial, appearance by humans add considerable weight to the speculation that preparedness plays a part in the development of BDD, particularly given the support for early development of this stereotype in children (Dion 1973). Certainly the complaint shares a considerable number of features with social phobia, since social activity is often avoided, for fear that the body attribute will offend others. As with anorexia nervosa, it can be suggested that in BDD these avoidances are secondary to the overvalued idea of bodily deformity. Diagnostically, the Diagnostic and Statistical Manual of Mental Disorders (DSM-IV) (American Psychiatric Association 1995) attempts to distinguish BDD, in which this idea although extremely fixed is amenable to rational argument, from Delusional Disorder, Somatic Type, in which the idea has reached delusional proportions and thus cannot be so modified. Clinically, this is a difficult distinction to make, given that fixity of ideation and amenability to persuasion are, by their nature, continuous rather than dichotomous. It has also been suggested that the term BDD be used exclusively for dissatisfaction with bodily *parts*, with the term Delusional Disorder, Somatic Type being reserved for overvalued ideas of delusional intensity about both body *parts* and bodily *functions*. In the current review, the expression 'bodily attributes' is used to imply both parts and functions for several reasons. First, in non-clinical populations, including disfigured people, dissatisfaction is expressed both with appearance and with function. Dropkin (1989) has suggested that it is possible to identify two separate scales relating to the severity of disfigurement and disturbance of function, but her study is flawed by the rating of functional disturbance by nurses, rather than by the patients themselves. Whilst it seems intuitively that form and function might well be separate dimensions and therefore amenable to separate rating, the two issues are often difficult to disentangle clinically, particularly where appearance and function are closely linked (Newell 1991). It is also worth remembering that appearance is itself a function, that of social expression of the self. Second, Marks and Mishan (1988) and Newell and Shrubb (1994) have argued that individuals who fear that they smell from halitosis, body odour or flatus are simply reflecting an overvalued idea regarding the body's ability to offend others via a sensory modality other than sight. Older studies (e.g. Beary and Cobb 1981), as well as the Marks and Mishan (1988) and Newell and Shrubb (1994) papers, have included such patients in their series, and used similar treatment approaches to those used with people having a concern over bodily appearance, with similar levels of success, indicating that the modality debate in BDD may be unimportant for treatment. Finally, Newell and Shrubb (1994) have noted that, with regard to bodily functions, there is no non-psychotic diagnosis equivalent to Delusional Disorder, Somatic Type in the same way that BDD is said to represent such an alternative in the case of body parts. Whilst hypochondriasis is a contender, it should be noted that, unlike hypochondriacs, individuals who claim offensive bodily functions do not necessarily claim illness. In view of this, it is concluded here that BDD represents complaints and fears that some bodily attribute (part *or* function) is offensive to others. This fear drives a series of behavioural avoidances (principally of social contact and exposing the body part assumed to be offensive) and excesses (such as checking rituals, repeated washing, wearing of excessive make-up) which handicap the person's life in a manner similar to social phobia and obsessive compulsive disorder, but with an overvalued idea related to body image similar to that in anorexia. For an examination of a fear–avoidance model of body image disturbance, it is probably best to retain as inclusive a definition as possible, to include disturbances of body image in which the sufferer expresses dissatisfaction with, and displays fears associated with, appearance, function, or both.

An expanding body of work supports the usefulness of a cognitive-behavioural approach to BDD, addressing both behavioural avoidance and the overvalued idea. The earliest accounts of successful behavioural treatment for BDD date from a single case report by Munjack (1978) using systematic desensitisation, and a small case series by Beary and Cobb (1981) using a variety of behavioural approaches, whilst Marks and Mishan (1988) reported success for exposure therapy in a study of five patients. The exposure treatment used was derived from work with phobic patients, and involved BDD sufferers deliberately entering situations which had previously been avoided because of what clients believed to be the reactions of others to their supposed deformities. However, patients in the Marks and Mishan (1988) study consumed many hours of therapist time, and recovery was incomplete in some cases. Moreover, several individuals had concurrent medication, which may have contributed to their improvement with exposure therapy. Nevertheless, these studies, and those of Neziroglu and Yaryur Tobias (1993a, 1993b), indicated considerable promise for exposure therapy. The first accounts of an integrated CBT approach which addressed the issue of the overvalued idea directly are attributed in the Gournay *et al.* (1997) review to Newell and Shrubb (1994) and Cromarty and Marks (1995). Newell and Shrubb (1994) combined the exposure technique of encouraging clients to enter situations avoided because of their assumed deformity, with generation of coping tactics, primarily through a series of role-play exercises in which the client would argue *against* the overvalued idea with the therapist, who would argue that the client's worst fears of bodily impairment were, in fact, true. As part of this exercise, clients were required to research and present evidence which refuted their overvalued ideas of deformity. The Cromarty and Marks (1995) case study was essentially a replication of this approach. Results from these small studies indicated considerable clinical improvement, with relatively modest therapeutic input compared with the Marks and Mishan (1988) series. The promise shown in these studies was supported in a small randomised controlled trial by Gournay *et al.* (1997). Clients received a 12-session cognitive-behavioural intervention package employing exposure and elements of the technique introduced by Newell and Shrubb (1994), and were compared with a waiting list no-treatment control. Clients in the treatment group fared significantly better than controls at the post-treatment point on all measures, and showed improvement over time between pre- and post-intervention scores on five of the seven measures. Clients in the control group showed no such improvements. Although the Gournay *et al.* (1997) study lacked a follow-up, the magnitude of the treatment gains, coupled with the continuing improvement of the two Newell and Shrubb (1994) cases at up to 18 month follow-up, indicates promise for the CBT approach to BDD.

This cause for optimism is strengthened by the findings of Rosen *et al.* (1995) in a study of fifty-four female BDD sufferers which randomly allocated clients to CBT or no treatment. Clients in the active treatment group received eight 2-hour group sessions. These included an integrated BT package, with more marked emphasis on behavioural components of treatment than in the Gournay *et al.* (1997) trial. Clients in the active treatment group fared better than controls on all five measures employed, both immediately post treatment and at a 4 month follow-up.

However, although Rosen *et al.* (1995) excluded anorexics and bulimics from their study, they included mildly obese individuals and it is clear from an examination of the subgroups that a considerable number had primary concerns regarding weight and weight-related appearance. Most other studies have treated only those with concerns about specific bodily features or functions. Thus, the Rosen *et al.* (1995) group may well differ considerably from other BDD series. Nevertheless, taken together, these results represent an encouraging picture for CBT intervention with BDD.

Newell (1991), Newell and Shrubb (1994) and Gournay *et al.* (1997) have suggested that the approach taken with BDD sufferers might be extended to include those suffering from actual disfigurement – as noted in Chapter 3, the model of body image disturbance advanced in this text draws in part on clinical work with BDD. However, one commentator (Latham 1997) has noted that since the defining characteristic of BDD is the absence of such physical abnormalities, such extension of the approach should be cautious, whilst another (Newell 1997) has suggested that, in the light of the work of Rumsey (1983) and Robinson *et al.* (1996), both Gournay's assertions and, by implication, Latham's commentary, are too conservative.

An earlier controlled study (Butters and Cash 1987) demonstrated that a mixture of *in vivo* desensitisation, relaxation and cognitive therapy techniques to address body image difficulties in a non-clinical population achieved greater change in body image than in controls. This ability of a cognitive-behavioural intervention to effect changes in body image contributes to confidence in the effectiveness of such interventions where disturbed body image is a major feature, even where this disturbance does not amount to the grossly overvalued idea present in BDD. Similarly, Tarrier and Maguire's (1984) study of post-mastectomy patients, which demonstrated significant improvement after treatment, suggests that, particularly if avoidance is a major factor of the client's difficulties, the effectiveness of exposure-oriented approaches which emphasise confrontation of the disfigured area is not confined to psychiatric populations.

In summary, there are limits to the inferences that might be drawn from studies of eating disorder patients, BDD sufferers and social phobics to treatment approaches for disfigured people. The principal limit is the lack of actual disfigurement in these groups. However, if we examine the clinical features of the three patient groups, we may see they share anxiety and behavioural avoidance as major problems; in the case of social phobics and BDD sufferers, social avoidance and the fear of negative appraisal by others; in the case of BDD sufferers and many eating disorders, disturbance of body image. These features all appear to be present in descriptions of disfigured people. It may, therefore, be possible to argue that similar processes mediate the difficulties of all these groups, and that a cognitive-behavioural approach is likely to prove useful in addressing psychological difficulties following disfigurement or other threat to body image.

Direct attempts to test the cognitive-behavioural approach

In order to explore whether more direct evidence might be found to support a fear–avoidance interpretation of the processes involved in psychological disturbance following disfigurement (particularly in social situations), Newell and collaborators undertook a number of linked investigations of the model. These are presented in synopsis form in the remainder of this chapter, and interested readers are directed to the original papers for further details. In essence, these studies sought to answer, by a variety of means, the questions of whether disfigured people showed anxiety in social situations and whether this anxiety might be phobic. Since anxiety and phobic avoidance are at the heart of the fear–avoidance model, answers to such questions might provide evidence to support or contradict the model.

Four studies relevant to this text were undertaken and will be described. These were a survey of media-recruited facially disfigured people, a survey of plastic surgery ex-patients who had undergone facial surgery, a controlled trial of a cognitive-behavioural intervention for social difficulties following disfigurement, and a comparison between facially disfigured people and phobic patients. The rationale behind these studies was to investigate the features of psychological distress present in disfigured people, the prevalence of such features, the possible effectiveness of a treatment based on a fear–avoidance model, and the presence or otherwise of a direct correspondence with diagnosed phobics. Additionally, a new instrument to measure body image related to the face (the Facial Attitudes and Avoidance Checklist, FAAC) was validated, but this process is not described here. Likewise, the measure and the survey procedures were piloted on a group of dermatology outpatients, and this material is not reported. Interested readers may like to examine Newell (1998).

A broad range of measures was used across the studies: the FAAC, the Fear Questionnaire (FQ), the Social Adjustment Questionnaire (SAQ), the General Health Questionnaire (GHQ 12), and the Hospital Anxiety and Depression Scale (HADS).

Media-recruited questionnaire study (Newell 1998)

The rationale for this study was that, as a minimum criterion for a fear–avoidance model of social difficulties following facial disfigurement to be viable, we should expect disfigured people to report anxiety and avoidance in social situations. Requests for participants were made through a range of media outlets (newspapers, magazines, radio and television) and 420 requests for details were received. Completed questionnaires were received from 46 male and 197 females thus represented 58.33% of the original enquiries. Mean age of respondents was 47.10 years (range 17 to 83 years), and was 51.80 years for males and 46.11 for females. Full details of the study are given in Newell (1998).

As might be expected from a self-selected sample, results from the media-recruited sample showed higher levels of disturbance than either the pilot or plastic surgery groups, although the majority showed low levels of disturbance. In response to the FAAC, dissatisfaction with the face and envy of others for their facial appearance scored high, but considerable numbers of respondents also reported disturbance on almost every element of the scale. In particular, a substantial *majority* (77.68%) of respondents reported that their face was a barrier with others at least sometimes, with 42.48% reporting that this was *often, usually* or *always* a problem. Perhaps more significantly for a cognitive-behavioural account based on a fear–avoidance model of disturbance in facial disfigurement, responses to the four elements of the FAAC's face/others subscale (which measures concerns about the attitudes of others to one's facial appearance) related to behavioural avoidance all showed considerable levels of difficulty. Some 29.06% of respondents reported avoiding walking in the street because of facial appearance at least *sometimes*, whilst 53.19% avoided social situations, 40.34% avoided sexual intercourse and 36.91% avoided certain clothes to a similar frequency. Moreover, 30.80% avoided looking at their own face at least *often*. Mean scores approached clinical levels of severity on the social phobia subscale of the FQ, and 25% of the group reached clinical severity on all subscales but the agoraphobia subscale. In response to the SAQ, only the social leisure subscale mean approached clinical severity, with 25% of respondents scoring 6/8 or more, although 25% of respondents scored 4/8 or more on the work subscale. Responses to the GHQ indicated some 114/233 cases, even using the stringent criterion for casehood chosen in this study. Responses to the HADS were particularly interesting from the viewpoint of a fear–avoidance approach to disturbance following facial disfigurement. Although the numbers of cases of both anxiety and depression were considerable, it is important to note that anxiety was far more frequently reported. Indeed, the *majority* of respondents attained scores indicating mild, moderate or severe anxiety on the HADS anxiety scale. These results, in a self-selected group, cannot be generalised as indicators of prevalence of difficulties amongst disfigured people. However, they do show the nature of the particular *patterns* of disturbance when it occurs. There is a marked tendency for these difficulties to involve social situations. Avoidance and anxiety are the most frequent features, lending support to the fear–avoidance formulation of psychological disturbance following facial disfigurement. Males and females were not different from each other on the majority of scales, but there were differences between respondents according to cause of disfigurement. Thus, those suffering disfigurement as the result of a skin complaint scored higher on the FAAC face/self subscale, the FQ problem severity subscale and the SAQ social leisure subscale than those disfigured following accident or injury, and higher on the FQ problem severity subscale, the GHQ and the HADS depression subscale than those disfigured from birth. Those disfigured from surgery scored higher on the SAQ work subscale than those disfigured from birth and from accident or injury, and higher on the SAQ home management subscale than those disfigured from birth. In general, therefore, those disfigured from skin complaint or surgery appear to suffer more psychological difficulty than those disfigured from birth, and more than those disfigured from accident or injury, although these categories are, of course, very broad, and may hide many differences between particular causes of disfigurement. Some of the differences found here may provide support for the cognitive-behavioural model, since people disfigured from birth may have more chance to habituate to anxiety in social situations.

A series of correlations were examined between the FAAC and the various measures of psychological distress and behavioural avoidance, and modest but statistically significant correlations were found in eighteen of twenty tests. Thus, there appears to be correspondence between attitudinal and behavioural aspects of body image concerning the face (measured by the FAAC) and the broad range of psychological disturbances measured by the other scales, including measures of phobic avoidance. These findings provide support for the fear–avoidance model of increased psychological difficulty following disfigurement, which asserts that disturbed body image, psychological distress, anxiety and avoidance (particularly in social situations) are associated. Responses to an open-ended question (Table 7.1) revealed a considerable range of tactics employed to hide the face, supporting the assertion from the fear–avoidance model that disturbance and the use of avoidance tactics are connected.

Survey of plastic surgery ex-patients (Newell 2000)

Forty male and sixty-two female plastic surgery ex-patients were successfully recruited from the medical records of two plastic surgeons. They represented 41.8% of the 251 ex-patients originally contacted. Mean age of respondents was 44.51 years (range 17 to 73 years), and was 49.93

Table 7.1 Media group avoidance tactic

Tactic	Number
Avert affected side	44
Use heavy make-up	10
Use hair as camouflage	14
Avoid eye contact	12
Wear beard	3
Wear glasses/sunglasses	7
Cover face with hand	25
Avoid strong lights	3
Avoid being photographed	7
Use clothing as camouflage	3
Other	12
No tactics stated	145

Source: Newell (1998).

years for males and 40.84 years for females. There were no differences between the age, sex and diagnosis of respondents and non-respondents. Participants received the same battery of questionnaires described in the media recruitment study.

As in the media study, levels of difficulty were generally low, but once again with considerable numbers of respondents showing difficulty. As might be expected, the general level of disturbance was lower than in the self-selected media-recruited sample. On the FAAC, high levels of dissatisfaction with the face and envy of others again occurred. Elements of the questionnaire battery concerned with social interaction showed greater disturbance than others. Caseness on both the GHQ and HADS were higher than the general population and higher than or similar to patient groups. It will be remembered, however, that the sample in this study are *ex-patients*, suggesting elevated levels of dysphoria amongst facially disfigured people. However, few individuals showed phobic avoidance of a severity requiring formal therapeutic intervention.

The comparison of males and females yielded different results from in the media-recruited group. Significant differences between the sexes were found in 7 of the 13 comparisons made. With one exception, all the significant differences reflected greater difficulty in females. The suggestion that females would show greater psychological difficulty than males receives modest confirmation in this sample, and offers limited support for the cognitive-behavioural model, which would expect socialisation of the two sexes to be different, and thus predict different responses to threats to body image.

One further source of comparison is of interest to the fear–avoidance model: between patients who had received surgery for cancer and those who had received surgery for revision of scarring from injury. It might, for example, be considered likely that the cancer group would be more psychologically disturbed as a result of having had to cope with a potentially life-threatening illness. Conversely, given that none of the subjects in the current study was currently receiving further treatment for cancer, the possible relief at having passed through the acute threat of diagnosis and treatment may have led to their being *less* disturbed than the scar revision group. In order to examine these possibilities, the diagnostic groups were arranged into two clusterings: cancer treatment (basal cell carcinomas, squamous cell carcinomas, malignant melanomas) and scar revision (scar revision, revision of road dirt tattooing). Other diagnoses were not included in the analysis. There were a considerable number of differences between the groups. Respondents in the cancer treatment group were significantly less psychologically disturbed according to their responses to the FAAC face/self subscale, the FQ social phobia subscale, FQ total phobias score, FQ anxiety depression subscale, FQ total problem severity score, the SAQ social leisure subscale, the GHQ, the HADS anxiety subscale and the HADS depression subscale.

Correlations between measures of psychological difficulty and phobic avoidance were, as in the media-recruited study, generally modest, again being significant on eighteen of twenty occasions. This increases our confidence in the results obtained in the media study. It may therefore be asserted that negative body image regarding the face is associated with higher levels of psychological avoidance and disturbance. These findings are again supportive of the assertion, based on the fear–avoidance model, that negative attitudes towards the face, fear and avoidance are related. The fact that the correlations with measures of behavioural avoidance apply equally to the body/others and body/self subscales of the FAAC indicates that this correspondence is not an artefact of the inclusion within the body/others subscale of items which specifically ask about such avoidances.

Controlled trial of a self-help leaflet for social difficulties following disfigurement (Newell and Clarke 2000)

Participants were 106 respondents to the questionnaire studies. They were randomly allocated to receive a 17-page leaflet either immediately after return of their initial questionnaire or 3 months later, and were followed up at the 3 month point. The leaflet focused on anxiety and avoidance in social situations and offered advice on cognitive-behavioural lines, particularly emphasising exposure principles (Marks 1987). Participants were selected if they achieved a cut-off score of 3/8 or more on the FQ global problem severity subscale. Thirty-four participants from the treatment group (six males, twenty-eight females) and thirty-six from the control group (five males, thirty-one females) returned follow-up questionnaires at the 3 month follow-up point, a response rate of 66%.

At follow-up, participants in the treatment group fared significantly better than controls according to the SAQ social leisure subscale, the HADS anxiety subscale and the HADS depression subscale. The first two of these scales may be considered as important tests of the fear–avoidance model because of their emphasis on socially phobic avoidance and anxiety respectively. Six further measures did not show differences. Of these, the social phobia scale was a key measure of social anxiety. On balance, there is support from this study both for a cognitive-behavioural approach to the social difficulties of disfigured people and for the fear–avoidance model of body image disturbance.

Comparison of facially disfigured people with phobic patients (Newell and Marks 2000)

The study group consisted of two groups. Phobic patients were 27 male and 39 female agoraphobic patients and 28 male and 40 female social phobic patients from whom anonymised data were obtained from a computer database held at the Maudsley Hospital, London. The facially disfigured participants were twenty-five male and eighty-seven female participants in the studies described above. Participants from this group were selected for comparison with phobic patients on the basis of a global problem score of 4 or more, in order to ensure a similar level of difficulty to the phobic patients, and compared according to their scores on the FQ agoraphobia, social phobia and anxiety/depression subscales. The rationale for the use of the 4/8 cut-off is described in Newell and Marks (2000), which also gives full details of this study.

The results indicated that people with facial disfigurement with global problem severity of clinical proportions demonstrate similar levels of socially phobic and agoraphobic avoidance to social phobic patients but higher levels of social avoidance and lower levels of agoraphobic avoidance than agoraphobic patients. This resemblance between socially phobic patients and facially disfigured people offers general support for a fear–avoidance model of psychological difficulty following disfigurement, since phobias are believed to be caused and maintained by fear and avoidance (Marks 1987), and specific support for the suggestion that the social difficulties faced by disfigured people are, in those who report psychological distress, socially phobic in nature. Facially disfigured people who experience psychological distress do not, however, resemble agoraphobic patients. The anxiety/depression subscale showed no differences between facially disfigured people and either phobic group, but power to detect differences between the groups according to this subscale was slightly low, and so conclusions from this similarity should be drawn with caution.

Summary of support for the fear–avoidance model from the above studies

If a fear–avoidance model of psychological disturbance following disfigurement is to prove viable as a way of examining and addressing this disturbance, we might expect to find a number of components to sufferers' experiences. First, it is a prerequisite that their difficulties contain a major component of anxiety, since this is a necessary component of any fear–avoidance model. Second, that anxiety should be more than that experienced by the general population, since *some* level of anxiety might be expected in anyone, regardless of the presence or otherwise of disfigurement. Third, there should be evidence of behavioural avoidance linked to anxiety. Fourth, disfigured people's difficulties should respond to a cognitive-behavioural approach based upon exposure principles, since this approach is known to be effective in addressing fear and avoidance (as in phobias). Fifth, those who report psychological difficulties should resemble socially phobic patients. Over and above this, the model also predicts that different groups of individuals might respond differently to disfigurement, on the basis of different life experiences prior to disfigurement. The effects of gender and cause of disfigurement may be fruitful avenues to investigate.

Before a summary of the extent of the evidence from the empirical studies described above is given, it should be noted that this might usefully be set in the context of some of the indirect evidence cited earlier. Disfigured individuals in qualitative studies have repeatedly described social difficulties, anxiety and avoidance, although the nature of these studies makes it impossible to generalise to disfigured individuals as a whole. Moreover, possible connections between these three elements of difficulty are rarely explicitly drawn and the construction of the studies makes it impossible to draw causal inference. Treatment studies of psychiatric populations with social avoidance, fear of negative appraisal and body image disturbance (social phobics, people with eating disorders and with body dysmorphic disorder) indicate that a cognitive-behavioural approach is effective, once again suggesting that fear and avoidance are major issues in these complaints. It is, however, a matter of debate how far it is permissible to generalise from these groups to disfigured people, unless it can be shown that they share characteristics important in the genesis and maintenance of their respective difficulties.

However, the four empirical studies of disfigured people described here appear to offer evidence to suggest that anxiety and avoidance are features of psychological difficulty in disfigurement; that anxiety occurs at greater frequency than in the population as a whole; that the psychological difficulties found are addressed with considerable effect by a cognitive-behavioural intervention based on the fear–avoidance model; and that disfigured people with psychological difficulties resemble socially phobic patients. Moreover, there is some suggestion from the data that different subgroups report different levels of disturbance in a way consistent with the fear–avoidance model.

From both the media-recruited and plastic surgery ex-patients surveys, it is clear that considerable avoidance takes place, as measured by the FAAC, the FQ and the FAQ. The last two of these measures specifically link avoidance with anxiety in the situations described. Moreover, avoidance of *social* situations is the most frequently described form of avoidance. High levels of general anxiety are also recorded, and, where it is possible to compare these validly with the general population (in the plastic surgery sample), are higher. Furthermore, examination of correlations between the FAAC and general measures of anxiety and avoidance suggests that less positive attitudes to the face (indicating disturbed body image) are associated with greater avoidance and anxiety. Thus, the nature of the disturbances suffered, their raised frequency and their association with disturbed body image are supportive of the fear–avoidance model.

Further support is provided by the treatment study, since treated individuals fared better than untreated ones, using an approach predicated on a fear–avoidance formulation of their difficulties. Although treatment gains were modest, the treatment input was likewise small (administration of a self-help leaflet), whilst the minimal nature of the intervention reduces the risk of an attention placebo effect accounting for the improvement. The fact that participants improved with even this minimal intervention suggests that the assumption underlying the treatment (that exposure to feared situations leads to a diminution of fear amongst disfigured people) is correct, and that such fear and avoidance are the mediating elements in the psychological difficulties of this group of disfigured people. The role of avoidance is further supported by the finding that disfigured people with psychological difficulties appear similar to diagnosed social phobics, according to a standard measure. Taken together, these findings point to the central role of fear and avoidance in influencing social difficulties related to threats to body image, regardless of the *actual* behaviour of others towards disfigured people.

Finally, there is some support for the notion that different life experiences may lead to different reactions to disfigurement, at least with regard to gender, cause of disfigurement and diagnosis. Women appear to fare less well than men when level of disturbance is slight across the whole sample, although this finding does not hold true when larger numbers suffer considerable disturbance, as in the media-recruited sample. We might speculate with regard to the different emphasis placed in our society on appearance in men and women.

The examination of different perceptions and behaviours according to cause of disfigurement is potentially important for two reasons. A fear–avoidance model of psychological distress following disfigurement suggests that different causes of disfigurement might lead to different patterns of difficulty, since they would contribute differently to elements of the model outlined in Chapter 3. For example, disfigurement from birth might lead to greater opportunities for habituation than traumatic or surgical disfigurement occurring later in life. By contrast, a remitting complaint, such as a skin disorder, might lessen such opportunities. It will be recalled that the skin complaint group in the media-recruited study did, indeed, generally show greater disturbance. Both disfigurement from birth and disfigurement from accident/injury respondents showed consistently better adjustment across a range of measures than people disfigured from skin disease or surgery, whenever such differences were present.

It may be speculated that the consistent finding of less disturbance amongst people disfigured from birth can be accounted for by a fear–avoidance model, since these individuals will have had more opportunity to habituate to the responses of others to them, and to their anxiety responses to the situations where such responses occur, although this assertion is somewhat weakened by the finding of no differences between the subgroup responses to the phobia subscales of the FQ, or the HADS anxiety subscale. The finding of less disturbance following accident/injury is not readily explicable in terms of the fear–avoidance model. The greater disturbance experienced by the skin complaint group may be explicable in terms of habituation, since skin complaints are often remitting complaints, where the sufferer has less time to become habituated to their appearance and its consequences before the complaint remits, only to return again. Clearly this interpretation is speculative, but it offers tentative support for a fear–avoidance model of disturbance following disfigurement, in the form of disturbed body image (as measured by the FAAC face/other), avoidance and general dysphoria.

In conclusion, the broad range of evidence in the four empirical studies described here supports a fear–avoidance interpretation. Moreover, there is some contextual support from studies of difficulties other than disfigurement. Whilst more work is needed, taken together these findings might be thought to offer sufficient evidence to offer some recommendations for clinical practice in addressing the difficulties which attend disfigurement and threats to body image, particularly given that empirical evidence in this field is thin on the ground. The final chapter explores the implications of the fear–avoidance model for intervention in psychological difficulty following disfigurement at the level of prevention, general education after disfigurement and intervention once psychological disturbance has been experienced.

Key further reading

Newell, R. and Shrubb, S. (1994) Attitude change and behaviour therapy in body dysmorphic disorder: two case reports. *Behavioural and Cognitive Psychotherapy* 22, 163–9.

Gournay, K., Veale, D. and Walburn, J. (1997) Body dysmorphic disorder: pilot randomized controlled trial of treatment; implications for nurse therapy research and practice. *Clinical Effectiveness in Nursing* 1(1), 38–43.
Two studies which suggest the role of treatments which have proved effective in BDD in addressing the difficulties of disfigured people.

Newell, R. (1999) Altered body image: a fear–avoidance model of psychosocial difficulties following disfigurement. *Journal of Advanced Nursing* 30(5), 1230–8.

Newell, R. (2000) Psychological difficulties amongst plastic surgery ex-patients following surgery to the face: a survey. *British Journal of Plastic Surgery* 53, 386–92.

Newell, R. and Clarke, M. (2000) Evaluation of a self-help leaflet in treatment of social difficulties following facial disfigurement. *International Journal of Nursing Studies* 37, 381–8.

Newell, R. and Marks, I.M. (2000) Phobic nature of social difficulty in facially disfigured people. *British Journal of Psychiatry* 176, 177–81.
These papers contain complete accounts of the empirical studies described in this chapter.

Chapter 8

Treatment implications of the cognitive-behavioural approach

Given that the cognitive-behavioural approach to client difficulties is a well-supported system of intervention, and since the fear–avoidance model of adaptation and disturbance following threat to body image is derived in part from this treatment system, it is not surprising that the model has immediate implications for interventions with patients. The previous chapter has demonstrated a number of sources of support for the fear–avoidance model, and it is argued that, in a field where evidence is often difficult to come by, these sources of support, along with the *general* effectiveness of cognitive-behavioural approaches to client difficulties, offer a tentative but viable basis from which to suggest potentially effective interventions which nurses can undertake with clients who are facing a threat to the integrity of their body image. The involvement of social distress and avoidance in body image disorder and disfigurement, and the acknowledged success of cognitive-behaviour therapy (CBT) in addressing such social distress (Fonagy and Roth 1996), add to the evidence for the potential viability of such an approach. This chapter presents a range of suggestions for intervention, within the context of treatment of emerging difficulties following disfigurement, general education (for example, around the time of surgery) and prevention.

The problem of body image disturbance is potentially vast. For example, Partridge *et al.* (1994) estimate the number of people suffering facial disfigurement at a level likely to be regarded as disabling as 250,000. Clearly, this does not include those suffering from 'invisible' threats to body image, such as the removal of internal organs. Given the findings of Wallace (1988), it is unlikely that many disfigured people will be in contact with psychological services, even though numerous researchers note that the level of handicap can be severe in a small but significant subgroup of sufferers. There is thus a need for intervention at a range of levels: specific interventions, preparation and general advice, and prevention. The fear–avoidance model, used in conjunction with an awareness of the areas of functioning likely to be affected (see, for example, Macgregor (1951), Rumsey (1983), Partridge (1990), Price (1990a, 1990b), Newell (1998)), leads to an approach which is potentially valuable across all these levels.

Cognitive-behavioural intervention for people experiencing difficulties following disfigurement

For individuals experiencing severe difficulties with body image disturbance and its associated behavioural avoidances and social difficulties, the fear–avoidance model and the cognitive-behavioural approach in general possess considerable advantages, as we have noted throughout this book. Dealing with complex cases of this kind is generally regarded as the role of specialist therapists – usually psychologists, nurses and psychiatrists who have undertaken specialist training in this approach. Newell and Dryden (1991) provide a readable general introduction to the cognitive-behavioural approach, whilst Marks (1987) presents an extensive review of the effectiveness of the approach in general and of exposure therapy in particular, and Richards and McDonald (1990) provide a good practical introduction. A detailed discussion of treatment is beyond the scope of this chapter, but the contention that only those specially trained in the cognitive-behavioural approach during lengthy post-registration education can successfully engage with disfigured people experiencing psychological difficulties is hard to justify. For one thing, specialist cognitive-behavioural intervention is in very short supply, whilst many nurses in specialist roles (e.g. head and neck nurses, breast care nurses) have not only developed considerable experience and training in interpersonal skills but may wish to encompass counselling roles in their repertoire of interventions. Given the success of CBT when compared with the more usual 'non-directive' forms of counselling (Fonagy and Roth 1996), the inclusion of cognitive-behavioural skills in the work of such specialist nurses should be greatly encouraged. Where available, supervision from someone experienced and trained in these skills will greatly enhance the learning of the nurse beginning to work from a cognitive-behavioural perspective. However, it should not be forgotten that CBT has been offered via self-help books, leaflets and even computer programs (Ghosh et al. 1984; Ghosh and Marks 1987), as well as by lay groups, with considerable success. It seems there is much that can be achieved, even without specialist training. Effective intervention will be likely to include the following elements:

- a detailed assessment
- a clearly explained rationale for CBT
- clearly defined goals
- a plan of treatment involving:
  - negotiated exposure to feared situations
  - tuition in social skills where these are lacking
  - tuition in challenging negative thoughts where these are thought to contribute to the maintenance of anxiety
  - involvement in treatment of family and friends
  - completion of 'homework' tasks by the client
  - generation of coping tactics and of rewards for successful completion of exposure tasks
  - identification and challenging of dysfunctional beliefs surrounding body image
  - planning to prevent relapse.

The cognitive-behavioural method of assessment

Cognitive-behaviour approaches to therapy generally give little emphasis to the concept of diagnosis. You will recall from Chapter 3 that CBT suggests that human difficulties are the result of genetic predisposition and environmental learning, in exactly the same way as are every other kind of human behaviour and experience. As a result, CBT is concerned, during assessment, with discovering the unique aspects of an individual's past learning which have led them to experience difficulties. This form of assessment is usually called *functional analysis* or *CBT assessment*. Unlike some other forms of therapy, the assessment process is often quite rigidly separated from other elements of treatment, and followed by a period of formal goal-setting with the client.

CBT assessment involves the therapists in investigating two basic elements of human experience: the three systems described by Lang (1971) and the contingencies associated with the client's difficulties. Although different variants of CBT depart from this approach somewhat, these central elements can generally be seen. Thus, CBT involves assessing elements of the client's autonomic/physical, behavioural and cognitive systems, and these systems are assessed antecedent to (before), during the behavioural episode, and consequent upon it. Moreover, such investigation is highly specific, in order to build a unique picture of the autonomic/physical, behavioural and cognitive features believed to be responsible for maintaining the client's difficulties. This has been described as assessment of ABCS (Newell 1994), because the therapist applies the approach shown in Table 8.1 to assessment of the client's main problem.

The 5 Ws approach (Richards and McDonald 1990) is useful in fleshing out the detail at each stage in this assessment (the sixth 'W' [Why] was a later addition by Newell 1994), so that precise details of what the client feels physically (with particular reference to the autonomic concomitants of anxiety), does (with particular reference to avoidance behaviour), and thinks (with particular reference to automatic negative thoughts which contribute to the maintenance of anxiety) may be gained. These details are important in helping the client to construct a treatment plan. In the case of a disfigured person suffering from difficulties in social situations we might, for example, expect a pattern similar to that given in Table 8.2 to emerge.

Table 8.1 The ABCS approach to assessment

(A)ntecedents
    (A)utonomic/physical
    (B)ehavioural
    (C)ognitive

(B)ehavioural event
    (A)utonomic/physical
    (B)ehavioural
    (C)ognitive

(C)onsequences
    (A)utonomic/physical
    (B)ehavioural
    (C)ognitive

(S)pecifiers
    What
    Where
    When
    Who with
    What do others do
    Why (what do you think causes the problem)
    [5(6) Ws]

    How long ago did episodes begin
    How do episodes affect the client's daily life

Source: Newell (1994).

Table 8.2 Assessment of a person with difficulties in social situations following disfigurement

(A)ntecedents (before being required to enter a social situation)
    (A)utonomic/physical (racing heart, increased respiration, sweating, nausea, muscular tension)
    (B)ehavioural (fidgeting, use of precautions and camouflage [e.g. medication, wearing special clothes or make-up], *actual avoidance of situation*)
    (C)ognitive (concentration on or rehearsal of the event to come, negative predictions, repeated negative self-statements ['people will look at me, people will pass remarks, I won't be able to cope'])

(B)ehavioural event
    (A)utonomic/physical (as above)
    (B)ehavioural (avoidance of eye contact, making conversation, standing in bright light, *not entering situation at all*)
    (C)ognitive ('people are staring at me, they think I look awful, I must leave')

(C)onsequences
    (A)utonomic/physical (diminution of above symptoms)
    (B)ehavioural (leave situation [earlier than planned])
    (C)ognitive ('what a relief, I should have been able to cope, I don't know how to face them again')

(S)pecifiers
    What (social gathering such as meals, evenings out, shopping)
    Where (friends' homes [best], pubs [worst], shops)
    When (frequency: at least daily; time of day: varies; duration: varies)
    Who with (friends [best with old friends], new people [worst], members of the public)
    What do others do (try to be friendly; look away; stare; pass remarks)
    Why (what do you think causes the problem):'I'm afraid of reactions of others'
    [5(6) Ws]

    How long ago did episodes begin (after getting out of hospital)
    How do episodes affect the client's daily life (feel upset all time; avoid shopping, meeting new people, going out alone, talking to others, wearing particular clothes, dating)

Rationale-giving and goal-setting

Following a careful assessment of this kind, the nurse is then in a position to offer a rationale for intervention and to agree treatment goals. For a full description of this process see Newell (1994) or Richards and McDonald (1990).

Rationale-giving

Offering a rationale for treatment is always important, in order to maximise the likelihood of adherence to clinical instructions. In the case of cognitive-behaviour therapy, where clients are asked to confront the things they fear, this process is particularly important, both ethically, since clients should know what they are letting themselves in for, and in terms of helping to generate adherence with instructions which require considerable commitment and resilience from clients. An adequate rationale for treatment should include:

- *A description of the nurse's initial formulation of the client's difficulties:* The nurse explains the role of avoidance in maintaining anxiety and increasing social handicap, the role of automatic frightening or negative thoughts in maintaining anxiety, and the role of exposure in decreasing anxiety.
- *A general description of the rationale underlying the nurse's proposed interventions for the problem:* The nurse explains in ordinary terms how exposure works (via the process of habituation through staying in feared situations until anxiety lessens), perhaps using examples from the client's everyday life, and explains how negative thoughts may be challenged by the client.
- *Specific examples of what is likely to be expected of the client and what the client can expect from the nurse:* The nurse stresses that feared situations will be entered, albeit in a gradual way, that anxiety will happen, but that this will gradually pass. The nurse and patient generate example situations together.
- *A prediction about the likelihood of success:* The nurse is positive but realistic, based on available evidence and clinical experience. The importance of measurement is stressed and the nurse seeks to enlist the client in a spirit of co-operative experimentation during the course of treatment to find out what works best with that particular client.

Goal-setting

Good goal-setting involves the nurse and client in agreeing goals which are:

- desired by the client
- indicative of change
- practically achievable
- representative of a range of activities.

In most cognitive-behavioural approaches, the goals are then formally measured by the client, giving a baseline against which to monitor change as it occurs during intervention.

Aspects of cognitive-behavioural intervention

Negotiated exposure to feared situations

Exposure has been a mainstay of cognitive-behavioural intervention for many years. Habituation, the basic principle behind exposure, was mentioned in Chapter 3. In practical terms, exposure therapy involves the nurse in drawing up with the patient a series of practical tasks which involve her in facing the feared situations in real life. The key component of this process is negotiation. The nurse seeks to help the patient towards identifying the optimum task they can attempt at any given stage in treatment. Ideally, this should be a task which involves the patient in entering a situation which gives rise to moderate anxiety and which is a step towards entering situations which the patient has identified as goals. The eventual aim is to enter these situations regularly and without difficulty. Some patients will be willing and able to withstand high levels of anxiety early in treatment, and this should be encouraged. However, there is little to be gained from attempting tasks which are beyond the patient's capacity to achieve at any given point, and the sensitive nurse attempts to gauge the extent of the patient's abilities at any given time. Three key elements should be emphasised both in the general approach to exposure as an intervention and at the start of any new task:

- The anxiety the patient experiences is normal and will pass provided they remain in the feared situation for sufficiently long. This is the basic principle behind exposure and is readily seen in such mundane situations as job interviews, learning to teach a class, meeting one's future in-laws for the first time and many other novel situations.
- The reduction in anxiety will occur more quickly the more frequently the relevant tasks are performed. Frequent exposure aids habituation and influences our expectations about subsequent events.
- It is not necessary to feel completely comfortable in a particular task situation before moving to the next most difficult task on the list. Exposure is about coping as well as comfort, since experience of coping alters our perception of our current and future ability to cope. It is necessary only to experience some diminution in anxiety (in order to prove to oneself the effects of habituation) and to

demonstrate to oneself that the level of anxiety in a situation is manageable (to prove to oneself that one can cope).

The tasks of exposure are ideally chosen by the patient, with the aid of the nurse in guiding them towards the optimally achievable task at a given time. Sample tasks for a facially disfigured person with difficulties in social situations might include:

- Shopping in empty, then near-empty, then crowded stores.
- Buying food at a takeaway, eating in a self-service restaurant, then a waiter service restaurant.
- Meeting old friends, going to a dinner party with friends, going to a dinner party at which new people will be present.
- Reducing the amount of make-up worn, ceasing to wear hats, dark glasses.

The key issue with the selection of exposure tasks is that they are relevant to the patient's areas of difficulty as identified at assessment.

Tuition in social skills where these are lacking

For many people, social skills are a set of behaviours which are learnt so unconsciously that they are never even labelled as having been learnt. They are simply part of the way we all interact – making eye contact at the right time, taking turns in conversations, starting and ending conversations, and so on. Frances Macgregor (1990) reminds us that, in the case of disfigurement, the basic equipment required for some of these important cues may be missing, for example where scarring diminishes the ability to move the eyes or to smile, or where surgery affects speech. The 'Changing Faces' approach emphasises the re-establishing of such abilities, and a number of leaflets are available. Apart from this actual absence of the physical ability to offer appropriate verbal and non-verbal cues, social reticence and fear of interaction may also lead to a situation where the skills of interaction are rarely practised, and resuming entering social situations, whilst important, may not be enough to re-establish social skills. The solution is formal practice of particular elements of skill which are lacking, whether in real life or via modelling and role play in comparatively safe situations where particular aspects of social performance can be practised over and over. Naturally, the nurse has a potential role to play in this, through both organising and participating in such situations. A number of relevant texts are given in the further reading section of this chapter.

Tuition in challenging negative thoughts where these are thought to contribute to the maintenance of anxiety

There is some debate in the literature regarding whether formal tuition of this kind contributes to improvement in phobic behaviour, and this debate is particularly important in the area of social phobia, which contains major elements of fear of negative appraisal by others. Some reviews suggest that this form of cognitive intervention adds to the efficacy of exposure-oriented treatments, although this additional benefit is relatively modest (Chambless and Gillis 1993). The process of disentangling the relative effects of these two components of treatment is problematic because (a) therapists offering exposure often also give considerable advice regarding the need to change negative thoughts and (b) cognitive therapies all involve behavioural experimentation which is similar in content to exposure. Regardless of this debate, it is almost certainly the case that some element of cognitive challenging and modification of fearful thoughts will be helpful, even if this challenging and modification is effective merely through the mechanism of enabling the patient to remain in the feared situation for sufficiently long for anxiety reduction to take place, thus enabling them to learn from direct experience that they are able to cope with such anxiety and that it passes provided they remain in the feared situations. The skilled nurse will want, as a minimum, to teach the patient to recognise the occurrence of repeated negative, anxiety-provoking thoughts and to generate some form of coping tactic (typically recognition of the role of the thought in contributing to anxiety and the generation of a coping thought to replace it). The systematic challenging of such thoughts is a formal system of therapy in its own right, and is beyond the scope of this chapter. Interested readers may wish to examine the relevant chapters of Hawton *et al.* (1989) as an introduction.

Involvement in treatment of family and friends

The support of family and friends is of great importance to the person seeking to overcome psychological difficulties, particularly in the cognitive-behavioural approach with its emphasis on practical tasks and confrontation of anxiety. Family and friends need an understanding of the nature of anxiety and its treatment, and of the role they themselves can play in assisting the patient. In particular, they need to be warned of the dangers in avoidance of feared situations, since families often believe they are helping the patient by, for example, excusing them from tasks and events which cause them distress. An explanation of the rationale for exposure treatment, the role of avoidance in maintaining anxiety and the role of family and friends in encouraging and participating in the confrontation of feared situations is essential at an early stage.

Completion of 'homework' tasks by the patient

Family and friends are particularly important in helping the patient with carrying out tasks related to their difficulties outside of treatment sessions. The nurse cannot be with the patient during all her attempts to enter the feared situations, and, indeed, it would almost certainly be antitherapeutic if she were to do so, fostering dependence. The patient and nurse will draw up a series of graded homework tasks which relate to the patient's difficulties.

Generation of coping tactics and of rewards for successful completion of exposure tasks

The nurse will be aware of the need to assist the patient in problem-solving when there are set-backs in treatment, such as times when the patient feels acutely anxious during an exposure session. This may involve generating coping thoughts (such as remembering that anxiety will pass over time), practising a relaxation exercise, or reminding herself of past successes. This works best when the nurse is able to bring forth such tactics from the patient's own repertoire of skills, rather than suggesting them to the patient herself.

We all need rewards to help motivate us, and this is particularly important when we are involved in potentially or actually frightening situations. Sometimes such rewards are intrinsic, such as the knowledge that we are working towards a desired long-term goal. At other times (particularly when that goal is quite distant or abstract) concrete rewards can be very helpful in keeping us on target. These can basically be of two types: we can either introduce some novel reward or we can structure our day so that things which we find rewarding occur after we have performed some task related to our eventual goal. So, for example, in writing this book, I might at the beginning of the day buy myself a bar of chocolate and allow myself a piece as a novel reward after each 500 words has been written. Alternatively, I might agree with myself not to have a cup of tea, a meal, a bath, or whatever, until so many words have been written. Since I find these everyday events rewarding, making them contingent on task performance has the effect of rewarding that performance, which in turn keeps me on target for the eventual goal. The application of self-reward for task performance during treatment is exactly the same procedure.

Planning to prevent relapse

This should occur from the beginning of treatment, and is part of the process, in cognitive-behaviour therapy, of assisting the patient to become their own therapist. Four elements are key:

- a thorough understanding by the patient of the processes of exposure, habituation and anxiety reduction (once again, this should be presented in everyday terms)
- an appreciation of the need to continue to enter the (previously) feared situations forever (skills which are not practised are often lost – I can't imagine how anxious I would feel if I had to go into an A & E department and perform as a clinical nurse tomorrow!), and to keep a careful check to see whether avoidances are creeping back
- a recognition that occasional difficulties are to be expected, are not catastrophic, and can be addressed by practising the skills learnt during treatment
- rehearsal, during treatment of potential problems in the future, and generation of appropriate responses.

Clinicians who are interested in pursuing the cognitive-behavioural approach further will find readable accounts in Marks *et al.* (1977), Richards and McDonald (1990) and Newell (1994).

Preparation for surgery and general advice

Appropriate education will be important in the context of preparation for surgery or medical intervention which is likely to result in a marked challenge to body image. This would include any visibly mutilating surgery, or any treatment which alters bodily appearance or function, such as radiotherapy, and also interventions which involve the loss of an internal organ or bodily function, since these interventions may also result in threats to body image. As in the case of treatment for those already experiencing difficulties, the cognitive-behavioural approach has much to offer. It is unfortunate that, whilst much has been written about patient education (see, for example, Viv Coates's (1999) text in this series) and preparation for surgical and other procedures, there is comparatively little which addresses preparation for changes in body image specifically. It is possibly comforting to speculate that this is because time is at a premium before and after surgery, or that clinicians genuinely believe their patients will cope (Holmes 1986). The alternative hypothesis, unfortunately, and one of which we should be acutely aware, is that clinicians, including nurses, are reticent about discussion of such matters, because of unfamiliarity or anxiety as a result of fears regarding the integrity of their own body image.

A precise description of what will happen to the patient is necessary before any procedure. In cases where a challenge to body image is to be expected, preparation should emphasise this element. From a cognitive-behavioural perspective, the description of the procedure and its physical consequences should be combined with an account of the likely psychological sequelae of changes in physical appearance, particularly where these changes are visible to others. Important information will include how the change may lead to fear, a desire to escape from, avoid or deny the change which has occurred. Wherever possible, as in formal cognitive-behaviour therapy, it is best if such information can be made relevant by relating it to the patient's own everyday experiences. This can also help patients to vent their own fears, and provide a forum for questions and advice. More particularly, examples may be found of situations or activities which might be avoided. The social context may be especially worth exploring. Some hospitals arrange for meetings with patients who have themselves undergone the procedures being discussed. Whilst potentially disturbing, these meetings may provide the opportunity for a potent form both of reassurance and of exposure to fear.

Preparation for the possible physical, psychological and behavioural changes that may occur is an important first step. Following this, an account of tactics patients might be able to use in addressing these potential difficulties themselves is likely to be useful, both in identifying coping tactics and in verbal rehearsal of these tactics. The aim of this part of any discussion will be to offer guidance specific to the difficulties foreseen or reported by the patient. The section earlier in this chapter on cognitive-behavioural approaches to intervention may be used as a general guide to this kind of preparation, but it may be wise to refrain from too much information, particularly prior to surgery, both because of the possible danger of overstating the potential difficulties and because the patient's ability to take in such information may well be limited by concentration on the prospect of the surgery to come. Rather, the general aim of such preparation may be to acquaint the patient with the idea that exposure to feared consequences leads to a decrease in distress. There is no need for complicated explanations, since most people have experienced the phenomenon of feeling anxiety in unfamiliar situations and the enormous, and also transitory, relief which comes from escape. Likewise, most people recognise, in their everyday life, that such escape tactics increase difficulty in the long run.

As a contrast, we have all experienced the examples of anxiety decrease over time mentioned in the section on treatment earlier in this chapter. This way of explaining the beneficial effects of habituation through exposure are probably a much more useful way of conveying the message of anxiety reduction over time to patients than appeals to conditioning or cognitive theories.

It is problematic that some level of avoidance is almost inevitable following surgery or other intervention. For example, the affected area may be covered in bandages, or the person may be unable to use the affected area. According to the fear–avoidance model, and according to cognitive-behavioural theory and the results of its treatments in general, this avoidance should be limited as far as possible, and patients should be encouraged to examine the affected area as soon as possible. For the sensitive nurse, this is a matter of negotiation with the patient. As in formal treatment, the job of the therapist is to involve the patient with the optimum level of exposure they can tolerate at any particular time. This involvement may include the formal agreement of a series of tasks to be performed, with the aim of giving the patient success in confronting anxiety from the beginning, and so increasing the likelihood of further such confrontation. The patient may also be offered some specific coping tactics, such as relaxation exercises or positive self-statements. For other patients, a much less formal approach may be valuable, and once again, it is the job of a sensitive nursing assessment to help in deciding the most useful approach. Common to all ways of engaging the patient, however, are four crucial components of the cognitive-behavioural approach: anxiety comes down as a result of confrontation (exposure); anxiety comes down more reliably the longer the exposure; anxiety comes down more the more frequent the exposure; reduction in anxiety generalises from the specific situations in which exposure is practised to other, similar situations.

It is worthwhile remembering that participants in the Newell (2000) treatment study improved with a minimal level of intervention. Even though many of them had been considerably handicapped for a number of years, they still made gains as a result of a simple self-help leaflet. In consequence, we may be fairly optimistic that many patients will respond positively to the general advice suggested in the paragraphs above. This level of intervention will be considered to be well within the expertise of most experienced nurses, particularly those active in fields relevant to disturbed body image. The provision of further self-help information will be valuable, and once again the leaflets and literature produced by 'Changing Faces' are a useful supplement to the advice of the nurse.

General self-help information such as Marks (1980) may also be suggested.

Prevention of psychological difficulties following a threat to body image

There is a pressing need for a greater understanding of the difficulties faced by people following threats to body image. In this connection, the role played by 'Changing Faces' is of considerable importance. In addition to the therapeutic work described elsewhere in this text, the group works to increase awareness of the challenges encountered by facially disfigured people. They do this through work with clinicians and researchers, through the media, and through their own publications, website and helpline. Much of their approach could be extended to other disfigurements and threats to body image. Nurses have the potential to contribute considerably to this consciousness-raising work. At one level, this may be formal, through the growing educational, primary preventative and public health roles of nursing, but nurses are also themselves both potential role models and potentially part of the problem. The stigmatising behaviour of members of the public towards disfigured people is well recorded. It is important that our profession does not contribute to this, and the education of the public is an important part of easing the lot of people with visible disfigurements in social situations.

More generally, although a number of self-help publications (e.g. Marks 1980) have brought cognitive-behavioural interventions to a wide audience, considerable education of the public regarding the role of cognitive-behavioural factors in the genesis and maintenance of psychological problems such as phobias is still required. The dissemination of this kind of information does not require particularly specialised knowledge if our aim is simply to create a broad awareness of the rudiments of the cognitive-behavioural approach to anxiety. Once again, everyday examples should suffice. The same is true of education of the public regarding disfigurement. For example, people may well be unaware that they stare at disfigured people, and of the distress this causes. As children, we were taught the social prohibition against staring at others, but it seems that this prohibition has been lost where disfigured people are concerned. It should, however, be relatively easy to reinstate. This kind of creation of an atmosphere amongst members of the public where, on the one hand, there is a general understanding of the need for confrontation of difficult situations and, on the other, an understanding of the need for (and right to) respect, privacy and anonymity in social situations is potentially important both to the general public and to those who go on to experience a challenge to their body image. Even if this importance is simply at a level of increasing awareness that difficulties based upon fear and anxiety are normal, widespread and, to an extent, understood and amenable to treatment, the nursing contribution could be significant.

The future of work with body image

The lack of research into facial disfigurement, its psychosocial sequelae and their treatment has been repeatedly noted in this book, and by previous commentators (Bull and Stevens 1981; Macgregor 1990; Houston and Bull 1994). It is surprising that there is also little systematic research with regard to body image generally, particularly given the importance placed on the psychosocial experiences of patients by nurses and other non-medical health professionals. Studies of treatment for disturbed body image are rare, outside the psychiatric literature. Given that the work of the Rumsey/Partridge group, and the fear–avoidance approach to treatment described in this chapter and Chapter 7, show potential, it is now important that further systematic investigation is carried out into these treatment forms. The results so far offer some support for the consideration of exposure therapy as a first-choice intervention with disfigured people experiencing psychological difficulties. Moreover, it may be argued that behavioural principles could usefully be explained to disfigured people at the time of disfigurement, as prophylaxis. This approach will, in itself, require rigorous testing. If the routine offering of cognitive-behavioural guidance to newly disfigured people proves of value, this might represent a major contribution to our management of disfigurement across a broad range of complaints. In consequence, the potential implications for service provision are far-reaching. With regard to the fear–avoidance approach, further specific tests of its predictions and assumptions would be useful, as well as treatment studies. More generally, all patient difficulties in which body image disturbance is an issue require continuing systematic examination.

One further important element worthy of study is the current level of psychological provision for disfigured people. Most writers in the field paint a dismal picture (Wallace 1988; Williams and Griffiths 1991) of patchy services and a general lack of consideration for psychological factors in disfigurement, and it has been noted that this latter trend has been present in the literature since its beginning. However, this is in striking contrast to the reaction of clinicians from all disciplines to the various studies carried out by Newell and collaborators described in Chapter 7. Anecdotally, two issues stand out in this connection. First, clinicians were generally concerned about their patients' psychological well-being, but lacked any strong sense of what they might do to address such issues. Where attempts were being made to address clients' psychological needs, this was generally being done in an ad hoc fashion, with little reference to any literature or other framework for action. Second, clinicians were generally enthusiastic about the current project and its possible implications for their patients. Their general feeling was that it was extremely unusual, and welcome, for a researcher to take an interest in their area of work. Interestingly, this last perception was echoed repeatedly by many participants in the Newell and collaborators studies. The congruence of their remarks with those of clinicians suggests the magnitude of the challenge of working with psychological care in facial disfigurement. In this connection, it is worth noting that there have been few published studies of empirical examinations of the need for psychosocial intervention following threat to body image. In terms of service delivery, we know the size of the task, and suspect that there is a massive shortfall in provision: a great increase in public awareness and concern will be required to produce the will amongst service providers to address this imbalance.

The volume of research into people's difficulties remains low, and we have little idea of the current level of service provision for these difficulties. Although the present author's own impression, anecdotally, is that there may have been some improvement in such provision since the published studies, this is based solely on personal contacts, which by their nature are with people interested in body image issues. There is a considerable need to get local initiatives into the public domain, both so that they can be submitted to scrutiny by peers and so that they may, where useful, act as beacons for good practice in the future. The work of Feber (1998), for example, serves as a good model of the introduction, validation and, crucially, dissemination of an approach to psychosocial difficulties, in this case with people with cancer of the larynx. Clinicians and researchers in the field need to expand the literature as a whole, but also to disseminate widely, both to clinicians and to people who have suffered a threat to body image themselves, in order to ensure the widest and most effective provision of services in an area where an appropriate therapeutic response is currently inadequately defined, described or delivered. With nurses being the major professional group in health care it seems inevitable that this task should fall on them. If we are to be taken seriously in our emphasis on a holistic approach to patient care, it is of paramount importance that we respond strongly to patients' needs in this most personal of areas of human experience.

Exercise

Consider the following questions:

- How far do issues of body image impact on your work?
- How far is the cognitive-behavioural approach consistent with your everyday experience of life?
- How far does this equip you to offer appropriate support to your patients?
- What level of involvement in addressing possible body image issues of patients do you want to have (e.g. general information-giving, specialist advice/therapy)?
- What further training, information and/or support do you need to equip yourself?

Key further reading

Hawton, K., Salkovskis, P.M., Kirk, J. and Clark, D.M. (eds) (1989) *Cognitive-Behaviour Therapy for Psychiatric Problems. A Practical Guide.* Oxford: Oxford University Press.
Classic general introduction to the specifics of the cognitive-behavioural approach to a range of client difficulties.

Richards, D.A. and McDonald, R. (1990) *Behavioural Psychotherapy: A Handbook for Nurses.* Oxford: Heinemann.
Practical guide for nurses wishing to explore cognitive-behavioural approaches.

Newell, R. (1994) *Interviewing Skills for Nurses and Other Health Professionals.* London: Routledge.
Similar to Richards and McDonald, but specifically aimed at the general nursing context, rather than mental health problems.

Trower, P., Bryant, B. and Argylle, M. (1978) *Social Skills and Mental Health.* London: Methuen.

Ellis, R. and Whittington, D. (1981) *A Guide to Social Skill Training.* London: Croom Helm.
Two very well-known texts covering social skills training.

References

American Psychiatric Association (1995) *Diagnostic and Statistical Manual of Mental Disorders, Fourth Edition, International Version.* Washington, DC: American Psychiatric Association.

Andreason, N. and Norris, A. (1972) Long-term adjustment and adaptation mechanisms in severely burned adults. *Journal of Nervous and Mental Disease* 154(5), 352–62.

Andreason, N., Norris, A. and Hartford, L. (1971) Incidence of long-term psychiatric complication in severely burned adults. *Annals of Surgery* 174, 785–93.

Baker, C.A. (1992) Factors associated with rehabilitation in head and neck cancer. *Cancer Nursing* 15(6), 395–400.

Bandura, A. (1977a) *Social Learning Theory.* Englewood Cliffs, NJ: Prentice-Hall.

Bandura, A. (1977b) Self-efficacy: towards a unifying theory of behavioral change. *Psychological Review* 84, 191–215.

Bandura, A. (1986) *Social Foundations of Thought and Action: A Social Cognitive Theory.* Englewood Cliffs, NJ: Prentice-Hall.

Barden, R.C., Ford, M.E., Jensen, A.G., Rogers-Salyer, M. and Salyer, K.E. (1989) Effects of craniofacial deformity in infancy on the quality of mother–infant interactions. *Child Development* 60, 819–24.

Barker, R.G. (1948) The social psychology of physical disability. *Journal of Social Issues* 4(4), 28–38.

Bar-Tal, D. and Saxe, L. (1976) Perceptions of similarly and dissimilarly attractive couples and individuals. *Journal of Personality and Social Psychology* 33(6), 772–81.

Beary, M. and Cobb, J. (1981) Solitary psychosis – three cases of monosymptomatic delusion of alimentary stench treated with behavioural psychotherapy. *British Journal of Psychiatry* 138, 64–6.

Beck, A.T. (1967) *Depression: Clinical, Experimental and Therapeutic Aspects.* New York: Hoeber.

Beck, A.T. (1976) *Cognitive Therapy and the Emotional Disorders.* New York: International Universities Press.

Beck, A.T. and Emery, G. (1985) *Anxiety Disorders and Phobias: A Cognitive Perspective*. New York: Basic Books.

Benson, P.L., Karabenick, S.A. and Lerner, R.M. (1976) Pretty Pleases: the effects of physical attractiveness, race and sex on receiving help. *Journal of Experimental Social Psychology* 12, 409–15.

Berman, J.S., Miller, R.C. and Massman, P.J. (1985) Cognitive therapy versus desensitization: is one treatment superior? *Psychological Bulletin* 97(3), 451–61.

Bernstein, N.R. (1976) *Emotional Care of the Facially Burned and Disfigured*. Boston: Little, Brown & Co.

Bernstein, N.R. (1982) Psychological results of burns. The damaged self-image. *Clinics in Plastic Surgery* 9(3), 337–46.

Blakeney, P., Herndon, D.N., Desai, M.H., Beard, S. and Wales-Seale, P. (1988) Long-term psychosocial adjustment following burn injury. *Journal of Burn Care and Rehabilitation* 9(6), 661–5.

Blumenfield, M. and Reddish, P.M. (1987) Identification of psychological impairment in patients with mild–moderate thermal injury: small burn, big problem. *General Hospital Psychiatry* 9, 142–6.

Bradley, B. and Mathews, A. (1988) Memory bias in recovered clinical depressives. *Cognition and Emotion* 2(3), 235–45.

Brewin, C. (1988) *Cognitive Foundations of Clinical Psychology*. London: Lawrence Erlbaum Associates.

Broder, H. and Strauss, R.P. (1987) Self-concept of early primary school children with visible or invisible defects. *Cleft Palate Journal* 26(2), 114–18.

Bronheim, H., Strain, J.J. and Biller, H.F. (1991) Psychiatric aspects of head and neck surgery. Part II: Body image and psychiatric intervention. *General Hospital Psychiatry* 13, 225–32.

Brown, B., Roberts, J., Browne, G., Byrne, C., Love, B. and Streiner, D. (1988) Gender differences in variables associated with psychosocial adjustment to a burn injury. *Research in Nursing and Health* 11, 23–30.

Brown, T.A., Cash, T.F. and Milulka, P.J. (1990) Attitudinal body-image assessment: factor analysis of the Body-Self Relations Questionnaire. *Journal of Personality Assessment* 55(1&2), 135–44.

Browne, G., Byrne, C., Browne, B., Pennock, M., Streiner, D., Roberts, R., Eyles, P., Truscott, D. and Dabbs, R. (1985) Psychosocial adjustment of burns survivors. *Burns* 12, 28–35.

Bruch, H. (1962) Perceptual and conceptual disturbances in anorexia nervosa. *Psychosomatic Medicine* 24, 187–94.

Bruchon-Schweitzer, M. (1987) Dimensionality of the body image: the body image questionnaire. *Perceptual and Motor Skills* 65, 887–92.

Bull, R. and Brooking, J. (1986) Does marriage influence whether a facially disfigured person is considered physically unattractive? *Journal of Psychology* 119(2), 163–7.

Bull, R. and Rumsey, N. (1988) *The Social Psychology of Facial Appearance*. London: Springer-Verlag.

Bull, R. and Stevens, J. (1981) The effects of facial disfigurement on helping behaviour. *Italian Journal of Psychology* 8, 25–33.

Butler, G. (1989) Phobias. In: K. Hawton, P.M. Salkovskis, J. Kirk and D.M. Clark (eds) *Cognitive-Behaviour Therapy for Psychiatric Problems. A Practical Guide.* Oxford: Oxford University Press.

Butler, G., Cunningham, A., Munby, M., Amies, P. and Gelder, M. (1984) Exposure and anxiety management in the treatment of social phobia. *Journal of Consulting and Clinical Psychology* 52(4), 642–50.

Butters, J.W. and Cash, T.F. (1987) Cognitive-behavioral treatment of women's body-image dissatisfaction. *Journal of Consulting and Clinical Psychology* 55(6), 889–97.

Carlisle, D. (1991) Face value. *Nursing Times* 16 October, 87(42), 26–8.

Cash, T.F. (1989) Body-image affect: gestalt versus summing the parts. *Perceptual and Motor Skills* 69, 17–18.

Cash, T.F., Winstead, B.A. and Janda, L.H. (1986) The great American shape-up. *Psychology Today* 20(4), 30–7.

Cassileth, B.R., Lusk, E.J. and Tenaglia, A.N. (1983) Patients' perceptions of the cosmetic impact of melanoma resection. *Plastic and Reconstructive Surgery* 74(7), 73–5.

Chambless, D.L. and Gillis, M.M. (1993) Cognitive therapy of anxiety disorders. *Journal of Consulting and Clinical Psychology* 61(2), 248–60.

Chang, F.C. and Hertzog, B. (1976) A follow-up study of physical and psychological disability. *Annals of Surgery* 183, 34–7.

Coates, V. (1999) *Education for Patients and Clients.* London: Routledge.

Cohen, C.G., Krahn, L., Wise, T.N., Epstein, S. and Ross, R. (1991) Delusions of disfigurement in a woman with acne rosacea. *General Hospital Psychiatry* 13, 273–7.

Conant, S. and Budoff, M. (1983) Patterns of awareness in children's understanding of disabilities. *Mental Retardation* 21, 119–25.

Crisp, A. (1967) The possible significance of some behavioural correlates of weight and carbohydrate intake. *Journal of Psychosomatic Research* 11, 117–31.

Cromarty, P. and Marks, I.M. (1995) Does rational roleplay enhance the outcome of exposure therapy in dysmorphophobia? *British Journal of Psychiatry* 167, 399–402.

Cumming, W.J.K. (1988) The neurobiology of the body schema. *British Journal of Psychiatry* 153 (Suppl. 2), 7–11.

Davidson, T.N., Bowden, M.L., Tholien, D., James, M.H. and Feller, I. (1981) Social Support and post-burn injury. *Archives of Physical Medicine and Rehabilitation* 62, 274–8.

Department of Health (1999) *A National Service Framework for Mental Health.* London: Department of Health.

Dewing, J. (1989) Altered body image. *Surgical Nurse* 2(4), 17–20.

Dion, K.K. (1973) Young children's stereotyping of facial attractiveness. *Developmental Psychology* 9(2), 183–8.

Doob, A.N. and Ecker, B.P. (1970) Stigma and compliance. *Journal of Personality and Social Psychology* 14(4), 302–4.

Dropkin, M.J. (1989) Coping with disfigurement and dysfunction after head and neck surgery: a conceptual framework. *Seminars in Oncology Nursing* 5(3), 213–19.

Dropkin, M.J. and Scott, D.W. (1983) Body image reintegration and coping effectiveness after head and neck surgery. *Journal of Social Otorhinolaryngological Head and Neck Nursing* 2, 7–16.

Dropkin, M.J., Malgady, R., Scott, D.W., Oberst, M.T. and Strong, E.W. (1983) Scaling of disfigurement and dysfunction in postoperative head and neck patients. *Head and Neck Surgery* 6(1), 559–70.

Edgerton, M.T., Jacobson, W.E. and Meyer, E. (1961) Surgical-psychiatric study of patients seeking plastic surgery: ninety eight consecutive patients with minimal deformity. *British Journal of Plastic Surgery* 13, 136–45.

Ellis, A. (1962) *Reason and Emotion in Psychotherapy*. New York: Lyle Stuart.

Ellis, R. and Whittington, D. (1981) *A Guide to Social Skill Training*. London: Croom Helm.

Faber, A.W., Klasen, H.J., Sauer, E.W. and Vuster, F.M. (1987) Psychological and social problems in burn patients after discharge. A follow-up study. *Scandinavian Journal of Plastic and Reconstructive Surgery* 21, 307–9.

Fairburn, C.G. and Cooper, P. (1989) Eating disorders. In: K. Hawton, P.M. Salkovskis, J. Kirk and D.M. Clark (eds) *Cognitive-Behaviour Therapy for Psychiatric Problems. A Practical Guide*. Oxford: Oxford University Press.

Feber, T. (1998) Design and evaluation of a strategy to provide support and information for people with cancer of the larynx. *European Journal of Oncology Nursing* 2(2), 106–14.

Feigenbaum, W. (1981) A social training program for clients with facial disfigurations: a contribution to the rehabilitation of cancer patients. *International Journal of Rehabilitation Research* 4(4), 501–9.

Festinger, L. (1957) *A Theory of Cognitive Dissonance*. New York: Row Peterson.

Field, T. and Vega-Lahr, N. (1984) Early interactions between infants with craniofacial abnormalities and their mothers. *Infant Behavior and Development* 7, 527–30.

Fonagy, A. and Roth, P. (1996) *What Works for Whom*. New York: Guilford.

Gamba, A., Romano, M., Grosso, I.M., Tamburini, M., Cantu, G., Molinari, R. and Ventafridda, V. (1992) Psychosocial adjustment of patients surgically treated for head and neck cancer. *Head and Neck* 14, 218–23.

Gardner, R.M. and Moncrieff, C. (1988) Body image distortion in anorexics as a non-sensory phenomenon: a signal detection approach. *Journal of Clinical Psychology* 44(2), 101–7.

Ghosh, A. and Marks, I.M. (1987) Self-treatment of agoraphobia by exposure. *Behavior Therapy* 18, 3–16.

Ghosh, A., Marks, I.M. and Carr, A.C. (1984) Controlled study of self-exposure treatment for phobics: preliminary communication. *Journal of the Royal Society of Medicine* 77(6), 483–7.

Goffman, E. (1963) *Stigma. Notes on the Management of Spoiled Identity.* Englewood Cliffs, NJ: Prentice-Hall.

Goin, J.M. and Goin, M.K. (1981) *Changing the Body. Psychological Effects of Plastic Surgery.* Baltimore: William & Wilkins.

Goldman, W. and Lewis, P. (1977) Beautiful is good: evidence that the physically attractive are more socially skilled. *Journal of Experimental Social Psychology* 12, 125–30.

Gournay, K., Veale, D. and Walburn, J. (1997) Body dysmorphic disorder: pilot randomized controlled trial of treatment; implications for nurse therapy research and practice. *Clinical Effectiveness in Nursing* 1(1), 38–43.

Gray, J.A. (1975) *Elements of a Two Process Theory of Learning.* London: Academic Press.

Gray, J.A. (1982a) *The Neuropsychology of Anxiety: An Inquiry into the Functions of the Septo-Hippocampal Region.* Oxford: Oxford University Press.

Gray, J.A. (1982b) A whole and its parts: behaviour, the brain, cognition and emotion. *Bulletin of the British Psychological Society* 38, 99–112.

Griffiths, E. (1990) More than skin deep. *Nursing Times* 4 October, 85(40), 34–6.

Hawton, K., Salkovskis, P.M., Kirk, J. and Clark, D.M. (1989) The development and principles of cognitive-behavioural treatments. In: K. Hawton, P.M. Salkovskis, J. Kirk and D.M. Clark (eds) *Cognitive-Behaviour Therapy for Psychiatric Problems. A Practical Guide.* Oxford: Oxford University Press.

Hay, G.G. (1970) Dysmorphophobia. *British Journal of Psychiatry* 116, 399–406.

Holmes, P. (1986) Facing up to disfigurement. *Nursing Times* 16 August, 82(34), 16–17.

Houston, V. and Bull, R. (1994) Do people avoid sitting next to someone who is facially disfigured? *European Journal of Social Psychology* 24, 279–84.

Hughes, J.E., Barraclough, B.M., Hamblin, L.G. and White, J.E. (1983) Psychiatric symptoms in dermatology patients. *British Journal of Psychiatry* 143, 51–4.

Jacobson, W.E., Meyer, E. and Edgerton, M.T. (1961) Psychiatric contributions to the clinical management of plastic-surgery patients. *Postgraduate Medicine* 29, 513–21.

Jaremko, M.E. (1986) Cognitive-behaviour modification: the shaping of rule-governed behaviour. In: W. Dryden and W.L. Golden (eds) *Cognitive-Behavioural Approaches to Psychotherapy.* London: Harper & Row.

Jourard, S.M. and Secord, P.F. (1954) Body size and body cathexis. *Journal of Consulting Psychology* 18(3), 184.

Kalick, S.M., Goldwyn, R.M. and Noe, J.M. (1981) Social issues and body image concerns of port wine stain patients undergoing laser therapy. *Lasers in Surgery and Medicine* 1, 205–13.

Kaplan, S.H. (1985) Patient education techniques used in burns centres. *American Journal of Occupational Therapy* 39(10), 655–8.

Kapp-Simon, K.A., Simon, D.J. and Kristovich, S. (1992) Self-perception, social skills, adjustment and inhibition in young adolescents with craniofacial abnormalities. *Cleft Palate – Craniofacial Journal* 29(4), 352–6.

Keeton, W.P., Cash, T.F. and Brown, T.A. (1990) Body image or body images? Comparative, multidimensional assessment among college students. *Journal of Personality Assessment* 54, 213–30.

Kleck, R. (1969) Physical stigma and task oriented interactions. *Human Relations* 22(1), 53–60.

Kleck, R.E. and Rubenstein, C. (1975) Physical attractiveness, perceived attitudinal similarity and interpersonal attraction in an opposite-sex encounter. *Journal of Personality and Social Psychology* 31(1), 107–14.

Kleck, R. and Strenta, A. (1980) Perceptions and impact of negatively valued physical characteristics on social interaction. *Journal of Personality and Social Psychology* 39(5), 861–75.

Kleck, R., Ono, H. and Hastorf, A.H. (1966) The effects of physical deviance upon face-to-face interaction. *Human Relations* 19, 425–36.

Koster, M.E.T.A. and Bergsma, J. (1990) Problems and coping behaviour of facial cancer patients. *Social Science and Medicine* 30(5), 569–78.

Lacey, J.H. and Birchnell, S.A. (1986) Body image and its disturbances. *Journal of Psychosomatic Research* 30(6), 623–31.

Landy, D. and Sigall, H. (1974) Beauty is talent: task evaluation as a function of performer's physical attractiveness. *Journal of Personality and Social Psychology* 29, 299–304.

Lang, P. (1971) The application of psychophysiological methods to the study of psychotherapy. In: A.E. Bergin and S.L. Garfield (eds) *Handbook of Psychotherapy and Behavior Change.* New York: Wiley.

Langer, E.J., Fiske, S., Taylor, S.E. and Chanowitz, B. (1976) Stigma, staring and discomfort: a novel stimulus hypothesis. *Journal of Experimental Social Psychology* 12, 451–63.

Lanigan, S.W. and Cotterill, J.A. (1989) Psychological disabilities amongst patients with port wine stains. *British Journal of Dermatology* 121, 209–15.

Lansdown, R., Lloyd, J. and Hunter, J. (1991) Facial deformity in childhood: severity and psychological adjustment. *Child: Care, Health and Development* 17, 165–71.

Latham, M. (1997) Commentary: Body dysmorphic disorder: pilot randomized controlled trial of treatment; implications for nurse therapy research and practice (Gournay, K., Veale, D. and Walburn, J.). *Clinical Effectiveness in Nursing* 1(1), 45.

Lazarus, R.S. (1966) *Psychological Stress and the Coping Process.* New York: McGraw-Hill.

Lefebvre, A.M. and Arndt, E.M. (1988) Working with facially disfigured children: a challenge in prevention. *Canadian Journal of Psychiatry* 33(6), 453–8.

Lethem, J., Slade, P.D., Troup, J.D.G. and Bentley, G. (1983) Outline of a fear–avoidance model of exaggerated pain perception – I. *Behaviour Research and Therapy* 21(4), 401–8.

Levitt, L. and Kornhaber, R.C. (1977) Stigma and compliance: a re-examination. *Journal of Social Psychology* 103, 13–18.

Love, B., Byrne, C., Roberts, J., Browne, G. and Brown, B. (1987) Adult psychosocial adjustment following childhood injury: the effect of disfigurement. *Journal of Burn Care and Rehabilitation* 8(4), 280–5.

McCrea, C.W., Summerfield, A.B. and Rosen, B. (1982) Body image: a selective review of existing measurement techniques. *British Journal of Medical Psychology* 55, 225–33.

Macgregor, F.C. (1951) Some psycho-social problems associated with facial deformities. *American Sociological Review* 16, 629–38.

Macgregor, F.C. (1979) *After Plastic Surgery: Adaptation and Adjustment.* New York: Praeger.

Macgregor, F.C. (1989) Social, psychological and cultural dimensions of cosmetic and reconstructive plastic surgery. *Aesthetic Plastic Surgery* 13, 1–8.

Macgregor, F.C. (1990) Facial disfigurement: problems and management of social interaction and implications for mental health. *Aesthetic Plastic Surgery* 14, 249–57.

Macgregor, F., Abel, T.M., Brut, A., Lauer, E. and Weissmann, S. (1953) *Facial Deformities and Plastic Surgery: A Psychosocial Study.* Springfield, IL: Thomas.

McKenna, H. (1997) *Nursing Theories and Models.* London: Routledge.

Malt, U. (1980) Long-term psychosocial follow-up studies of burned adults: review of the literature. *Burns* 6, 190–7.

Malt, U.F. and Ugland, O.M. (1989) A long-term psychosocial follow-up study of burned adults. *Acta Psychiatrica Scandinavica Suppl.* 355(80), 94–102.

Marks, I.M. (1980) *Living With Fear.* New York: McGraw-Hill.

Marks, I.M. (1986) *Behavioural Psychotherapy: The Maudsley Pocket Book of Clinical Management.* Bristol: Wright.

Marks, I.M. (1987) *Fears, Phobias and Rituals.* New York: Oxford University Press.

Marks, I.M. and Mishan, J. (1988) Dysmorphophobic avoidance with disturbed bodily perception: a pilot study of exposure therapy. *British Journal of Psychiatry* 152, 674–8.

Marks, I.M., Hallam, R.S., Connolly, J. and Philpott, R. (1977) *Nursing in Behavioural Psychotherapy.* London: Royal College of Nursing.

Martin, J., Meltzer, H. and Elliot, D. (1988) *Office of Population Censuses and Surveys Social Survey Division. Surveys of Disability in Great Britain, Report 1: The Prevalence of Disability among Adults.* London: OPCS.

Meichenbaum, D. (1977) *Cognitive Behavior Modification.* Morristown, NJ: General Learning Press.

Moore, P., Blakeney, P., Bromeling, L., Portman, S., Herndon, D.N. and Robson, M. (1993) Psychologic adjustment after childhood burn injuries as predicted by personality traits. *Journal of Burn Care and Rehabilitation* 14(1), 80–2.

Mowrer, O.H. (1960) *Learning Theory and Behavior.* New York: Wiley.

Munjack, D.J. (1978) The behavioral treatment of dysmorphophobia. *Journal of Behavior Therapy and Experimental Psychiatry* 9, 53–6.

Newell, R. (1991) Body image disturbance: cognitive-behavioural formulation and intervention. *Journal of Advanced Nursing* 16, 1400–5.

Newell, R. (1994) *Interviewing Skills for Nurses and Other Health Professionals*. London: Routledge.

Newell, R. (1996) Behaviour therapy. In: W. Dryden (ed.) *Developments in Psychotherapy*. Newbury Park: Sage.

Newell, R.J. (1997) Commentary: Body dysmorphic disorder: pilot randomized controlled trial of treatment; implications for nurse therapy research and practice (Gournay, K., Veale, D. and Walburn, J.). *Clinical Effectiveness in Nursing* 1(1), 44.

Newell, R. (1998) *Facial disfigurement and avoidance: a cognitive-behavioural approach*. Unpublished PhD thesis, University of Hull.

Newell, R. (1999) Altered body image: a fear–avoidance model of psychosocial difficulties following disfigurement. *Journal of Advanced Nursing* 30(5), 1230–8.

Newell, R. (2000) Psychological difficulties amongst plastic surgery ex-patients following surgery to the face: a survey. *British Journal of Plastic Surgery* 53, 386–92.

Newell, R. and Clarke, M. (2000) Evaluation of a self-help leaflet in treatment of social difficulties following facial disfigurement. *International Journal of Nursing Studies* 37, 381–8.

Newell, R.J. and Dryden, W. (1991) Clinical problems: an introduction to the cognitive-behavioural approach. In: W. Dryden and R. Rentoul (eds) *Adult Clinical Problems: A Cognitive-Behavioural Approach*. London: Routledge.

Newell, R. and Marks, I.M. (2000) Phobic nature of social difficulty in facially disfigured people. *British Journal of Psychiatry* 176, 177–81.

Newell, R. and Shrubb, S. (1994) Attitude change and behaviour therapy in body dysmorphic disorder: two case reports. *Behavioural and Cognitive Psychotherapy* 22, 163–9.

Neziroglu, F. and Yaryura Tobias, J.A. (1993a) Body dysmorphic disorder: phenomenology and case descriptions. *Behavioural Psychotherapy* 21, 27–36.

Neziroglu, F. and Yaryura Tobias, J.A. (1993b) Exposure, response prevention and cognitive therapy in the treatment of body dysmorphic disorder. *Behavior Therapy* 24, 431–8.

Noar, J.H. (1991) Questionnaire survey of attitudes and concerns of patients with cleft lip and palate and their parents. *Cleft Palate – Craniofacial Journal* 28(3), 279–84.

Novak, D.W. and Lerner, M.J. (1968) Rejection as a consequence of perceived similarity. *Journal of Personality and Social Psychology* 9(2), 147–52.

Orr, D.A., Reznikoff, M. and Smith, G.M. (1989) Body image, self-esteem and depression in burn-injured adolescents and young adults. *Journal of Burn Care and Rehabilitation* 10(5), 454–61.

Partridge, J. (1990) *Changing Faces: The Challenge of Facial Disfigurement.* London: Penguin.

Partridge, J. (1991) Staring prejudice in the face. *Nursing Times* 16 October, 87(42), 28–30.

Partridge, J. (1993) The psychological effects of facial disfigurement. *Journal of Wound Care* 2(3), 168–71.

Partridge, J., Coutinho, W., Robinson, E. and Rumsey, N. (1994) Changing Faces: two years on. *Nursing Standard* 18 May, 8(34), 54–8.

Pertschuk, M.J. and Whitaker, L.A. (1982) Social and psychological effects of craniofacial deformity and surgical reconstruction. *Clinics in Plastic Surgery* 9(3), 297–306.

Piff, C. (1985) *Let's Face It.* London: Victor Gollancz.

Piliavin, I.M., Piliavin, J.A. and Rodin, J. (1975) Costs, diffusion and the stigmatized person. *Journal of Personality and Social Psychology* 32, 429–38.

Porter, J.R., Beuf, A.H., Lerner, A. and Nordlund, J. (1986) Psychosocial effect of vitiligo: a comparison of vitiligo patients with 'normal' control subjects, with psoriasis patients and with patients with other pigmentary disorders. *Journal of the American Academy of Dermatology* 15(2), 220–4.

Price, R. (1986) Keeping up appearances. *Nursing Times* 1 October, 82(40), 58–61.

Price, R. (1990a) A model for body image care. *Journal of Advanced Nursing* 15, 585–93.

Price, R. (1990b) *Body Image: Nursing Concepts and Care.* New York: Prentice Hall.

Price, R. (1996) Assessing altered body image. *Journal of Psychiatric and Mental Health Nursing* 2, 169–75.

Pruzinsky, T. (1992) Social and psychological effects of major craniofacial deformity. *Cleft Palate – Craniofacial Journal* 29(6), 578–84.

Rachman, S.J. and Hodgson, R. (1974) Synchrony and desynchrony in fear and avoidance. *Behaviour Research and Therapy* 12, 311–18.

Rachman, S.J. and Wilson, G.T. (1980) *The Effects of Psychological Therapy.* Oxford: Pergamon.

Raza, S.M. and Carpenter, B.N. (1987) A model of hiring decisions in real employment interviews. *Journal of Applied Psychology* 72, 596–603.

Reich, J. (1969) The surgery of appearance: psychological and related aspects. *Medical Journal of Australia* 2, 5–13.

Reis, H.T., Nelzek, J. and Wheeler, L. (1980) Physical attractiveness in social interaction. *Journal of Personality and Social Psychology* 38(4), 604–17.

Rich, J. (1975) Effects of children's physical attractiveness on teachers' evaluations. *Journal of Educational Psychology* 67, 599–609.

Richards, D.A. and McDonald, R. (1990) *Behavioural Psychotherapy: A Handbook for Nurses.* Oxford: Heinemann.

Richman, L.C. and Eliason, M. (1982) Psychological characteristics of children with cleft lip and palate: intellectual, achievement, behavioral and personality variables. *Cleft Palate Journal* 19, 249–57.

Robinson, E., Rumsey, N. and Partridge, J. (1996) An evaluation of the impact of social interaction skills training for facially disfigured people. *British Journal of Plastic Surgery* 49, 281–9.

Roca, R.P., Spence, M.J. and Munster, A.M. (1992) Post-traumatic adaptation and distress among adult burn survivors. *American Journal of Psychiatry* 149(9), 1234–8.

Rose, M.J., Klenerman, L., Atchison, L. and Slade, P.D. (1992) An application of the fear avoidance model to three chronic pain problems. *Behaviour Research and Therapy* 30(4), 359–65.

Rosen, J.C., Reiter, J. and Orosan, P. (1995) Cognitive-behavioral body image therapy for body dysmorphic disorder. *Journal of Consulting and Clinical Psychology* 63(2), 263–9.

Rubinow, D.R., Peck, G.L., Squillace, K.M. and Gantt, G.G. (1987) Reduced anxiety and depression in cystic acne patients after successful treatment with oral isotretinoin. *Journal of the American Academy of Dermatology* 17(1), 25–32.

Rumsey, N. (1983) *Psychological problems associate with facial disfigurement.* Unpublished PhD thesis, North East London Polytechnic.

Rumsey, N., Bull, R. and Gahagan, D. (1986a) A developmental study of children's stereotyping of facially deformed adults. *British Journal of Psychology* 77, 269–74.

Rumsey, N., Bull, R. and Gahagan, D. (1986b) A preliminary study of the potential of social skills for improving the quality of social interaction for the facially disfigured. *Social Behaviour* 1, 143–5.

Russell, G. (1970) Anorexia nervosa: its identity as an illness and its treatment. In: O.W. Hill (ed.) *Modern Trends in Psychological Medicine.* London: Butterworth.

Salkovskis, P. and Kirk, J. (1989) Obsessional disorders. In: K. Hawton, P.M. Salkovskis, J. Kirk and D.M. Clark (eds) *Cognitive-Behaviour Therapy for Psychiatric Problems. A Practical Guide.* Oxford: Oxford University Press.

Samerotte, G.C. and Harris, M.B. (1976) Some factors influencing helping: the effects of a handicap, responsibility and requesting help. *Journal of Social Psychology* 98, 39–45.

Schilder, P. (1935) *Image and Appearance of the Human Body.* London: Kegan Paul.

Scott, D.W., Oberst, M. and Dropkin, M.J. (1980) A stress-coping model. *Advances in Nursing Science* 3, 9–23.

Secord, P.F. (1953) Objectification of word association procedures by the use of homonyms: a measure of body cathexis. *Journal of Personality* 21, 479–95.

Secord, P.F. and Jourard, S.M. (1953) The appraisal of body-cathexis: body-cathexis and the self. *Journal of Consulting Psychology* 17(5), 343–7.

Seligman, M.E.P. (1971) Phobias and preparedness. *Behavior Therapy* 2, 307–20.

Shakin Kunkel, E.J., Rodgers, C., Field, H.L., Snyderman, D.A., Woods, C., Zager, R.P. and Walker, M. (1995) Treating the patient who is disfigured by head and neck cancer. *General Hospital Psychiatry* 17, 444–50.

Shapiro, D.A. and Shapiro, D. (1982) Meta-analysis of comparative therapy outcome studies: a replication and refinement. *Psychological Bulletin* 92, 581–604.

Shaw, W.C. (1986) Comment: Applied psychological research in the clinical management of dental and facial deformity. *Human Learning* 5, 209–10.

Shaw, W.C., Humphreys, S., McLoughlin, J.M. and Shimmin, P.C. (1980) The effect of facial deformity on petitioning. *Human Relations* 33(9), 659–71.

Shuster, S., Fisher, G.H., Harris, E. and Binnell, D. (1978) The effect of skin disease on self image. *British Journal of Dermatology* 99, 18–19.

Sigall, H. and Landy, L. (1973) Radiating beauty: effects of having a physically attractive partner on person perception. *Journal of Personality and Social Psychology* 28(2), 218–24.

Sigelman, C.K. and Singleton, L.C. (1986) Stigmatization in childhood: a survey of developmental needs and issues. In: S.C. Ainley, G. Becker and L.M. Coleman (eds) *The Dilemma of Difference: A Multidisciplinary View of Stigma*. New York: Plenum.

Slade, P.D. (1988) Body image in anorexia nervosa. *British Journal of Psychiatry* 153 (Suppl. 2), 20–2.

Slade, P.D. (1994) What is body image? *Behaviour Research and Therapy* 32(5), 497–502.

Slade, P.D., Troup, J.D.G., Lethem, J. and Bentley, G. (1983) The fear–avoidance model of exaggerated pain perception – II. Preliminary studies of coping strategies for pain. *Behaviour Research and Therapy* 21(4), 409–16.

Smith, M.L. and Glass, G.V. (1977) Meta-analysis of psychotherapy outcome studies. *American Psychologist* 32, 752–60.

Snyder, M., Tanke, E.D. and Berscheid, E. (1977) Social perception and interpersonal behaviour: on the self-fulfilling nature of social stereotypes. *Journal of Personality and Social Psychology* 35(9), 656–66.

Soble, S.L. and Strickland, L.H. (1974) Physical stigma, interaction and compliance. *Bulletin of the Psychonomic Society* 4(2B), 130–2.

Starr, P. (1980) Facial attractiveness and behavior of patients with cleft lip and/or palate. *Psychological Reports* 46, 579–82.

Stavynski, A. and Greenberg, D. (1998) The treatment of social phobia: a critical assessment. *Acta Psychiatrica Scandinavica* 98(3), 171–81.

Tarrier, N. and Maguire, P. (1984) Treatment of psychological distress following mastectomy: an initial report. *Behaviour Research and Therapy* 22(1), 81–4.

Taylor, S. (1996) Meta-analysis of cognitive-behavioral treatments for social phobia. *Journal of Behavior Therapy and Experimental Psychiatry* 27(1), 1–9.

Trower, P., Bryant, B. and Argylle, M. (1978) *Social Skills and Mental Health*. London: Methuen.

Tucker, P. (1987) Psychosocial problems among adult burn victims. *Burns* 13(1), 7–14.

Ungar, S. (1979) The effects of effort and stigma on helping. *Journal of Social Psychology* 107, 23–8.

Walker, S. (1984) *Learning Theory and Behaviour Modification.* London: Methuen.

Walker, S. (1987) *Animal Learning.* London: Routledge & Kegan Paul.

Wallace, L.A. (1988) Abandoned to a social death. *Nursing Times* 9 March, 84(10), 34–7.

White, A.C. (1982) Psychiatric study of patients with severe burns. *British Medical Journal* 284, 465–7.

Williams, E.E. and Griffiths, T.A. (1991) Psychological consequences of burn injury. *Burns* 17(6), 478–80.

Williams, J.M.G., Watts, F.N., MacLeod, C. and Mathews, A. (1988) *Cognitive Psychology and Emotional Disorders.* Chichester: Wiley.

Wolpe, J. (1952) Objective psychotherapy of the neuroses. *South African Medical Journal* 26, 825–9.

Wolpe, J. (1958) *Psychotherapy by Reciprocal Inhibition.* Stanford: Stanford University Press.

Wolpe, J. (1978) Cognition and causation in human behavior and its therapy. *American Psychologist* 33, 437–46.

Worthington, M.E. (1974) Personal space as a function of the stigma effect. *Environment and Behavior* 6(3), 289–94.

Zimbardo, P. and Ebbeson, E.B. (1970) *Influencing Attitudes and Changing Behavior.* New York: Addison-Wesley.

Author index

Subject index